Endangered Hope

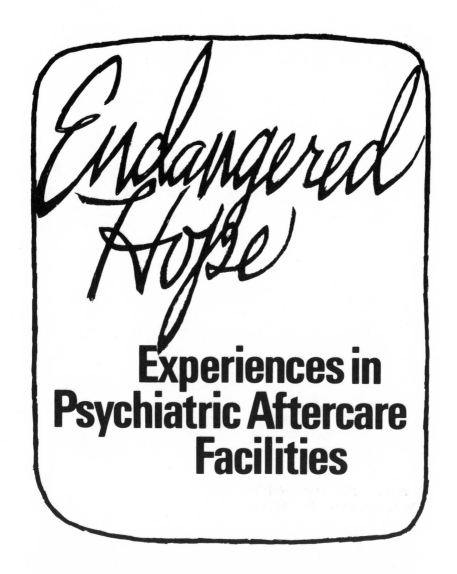

Endangered Hope

Experiences in Psychiatric Aftercare Facilities

David K. Reynolds and Norman L. Farberow

University of California Press

Berkeley · Los Angeles · London

1977

University of California Press
Berkeley and Los Angeles, California

University of California Press, Ltd.
London, England

CONTENTS

FOREWORD

It gives me great pleasure to write the foreword to this latest book by Dr. Reynolds and Dr. Farberow. I worked with them on several phases of their experiential research, including selection of the settings in which the research was conducted. I am familiar with the aftercare facilities and am acquainted with the sponsors, and with some of the posthospitalized residents about whom they report.

Dr. Reynolds characteristically approaches his anthropological studies not only by observing and evaluating a particular group but also by actually taking on the identity of a member of the group he is studying. He followed this procedure in an earlier research adventure (Reynolds and Farberow, *Suicide: Inside and Out,* 1976) in order to understand suicide in mental hospitals. And he has done it again in his concern to discover what takes place in the life of the discharged depressed person struggling to get well. His aim is to get into the role of such a person and actually to experience the feelings of depression. In fact, after the completion of a study it may require weeks for him to begin to feel once again like his former self. While it is always difficult, of course, to learn about the intimate pain and hurt that each person keeps locked up inside himself, Dr. Reynolds's findings do provide a close look into the individual's day-by-day existence and the impact the attitudes and behaviors of others have on him. For the sensitive person it is the careless gesture, the lack of consideration, and the seeming unawareness of other's feelings (the poor manners, if you will) which most deeply offend. The work of Reynolds and Farberow provides a core of solid material enabling family care sponsors and residential care personnel to become aware of growth-producing influences and negative elements that block the depressed person's movement toward wellness.

The authors offer pertinent recommendations for creating a more workable social support system for the person leaving the protective hospital setting. The idea of starting out in pairs or groups is worthwhile and entirely realistic. Our hospital staff has already had some success with pairs entering the community together, and we would be in complete accord with the thought of continuing and enlarging upon the practice.

A method of evaluating and grading the personnel of aftercare facilities according to special interests, talents, and abilities has been a badly neglected area. Although the problem is difficult and time-consuming, its solution would certainly be a major step toward ensuring the kind of environment that would encourage a return to good health. In considering sponsor candidates for developing after-care programs, I believe applicants are more aware of some of their own limitations than we may think. I would like to see a more intensive use of techniques that help the poorly equipped or poorly motivated candidates to screen themselves, if not at the point of application for sponsorship, at least when it becomes obvious that the assignment is beyond their capacity. Some sponsors, of course, are best equipped to operate simple programs geared primarily to meeting their patients' physical needs. There are always individuals who leave the hospital seeking only comfortable permanent residences. They need such sponsors and facilities. But it is the sponsor with the motivation and the talent to develop a genuinely therapeutic posthospital environment who is so badly needed.

I believe that some residential programs and family-care homes are run by imaginative people who would like to try different ways of helping but who hesitate for fear of failure or criticism. This group would, I think, be appropriate for the special assignment the authors mention, working with a small group of residents, organizing training projects in preparation for independent living, and the like. It is worth mentioning here that the facility's personnel as well as the successful resident who graduates from such a program should be given recognition as a means of acknowledging a job well done and as an inspiration for further effort.

These brief comments bring me to a point that the authors stress repeatedly: the critical need for more professional consultation.

Personnel who work with individuals struggling to get well carry a heavy load, and they know it. Far more often than we like to think they feel very much alone with the perplexity, the fear, and the discouragement evoked by this day-to-day struggle. Perhaps the most important message this study brings us is the immediate and imperative need for steady ongoing professional help for the personnel engaged in this serious, lifesaving, twenty-four-hour-a-day job.

Joseph T. Crockett, M.D., F.A.P.A.

Los Angeles, California

ACKNOWLEDGMENTS

Our thanks are owing to the residential aftercare operators and staff members who invited us to enter their facilities and to residents who shared their lives with David Kent and Helen Summers. They must, of course, remain anonymous so as to protect the confidences they revealed.

Without the cooperation of Dr. Joseph Crockett, Chief, Psychiatric Unit I; Veterans Administration Brentwood Hospital, social workers Keith Froehlich, Sharon Gallagher, and Shirley English; Rosa Maddox of Community Services, and psychologist Dr. David Wine, our study would have been extremely difficult, or perhaps even impossible.

We acknowledge gratefully the consistent support of Research Service, Veterans Administration Wadsworth Hospital Center, in providing time and encouragement for conducting the study.

Special recognition must go to Helen Sullivan, who invested time and insightful effort in living in one board-and-care facility.

Claudette Martin and Majda Andlovec contributed time and effort in typing the study.

To James Kubeck, who skillfully guided the manuscript through the editorial stages, and to Grace H. Stimson, who expertly edited the manuscript, we are grateful.

The views we present in this book are filtered through the lenses of our experiences and biases. To put the perspective of any aftercare residents in print, however, seems to us to be an important step toward improvement of living conditions, for both residents and staff, in these facilities. The settings have changed somewhat since the period in which our research was conducted. One facility has moved to another building. Others have had significant turnovers in staff and residents. All facilities have introduced changes as a result of our postresearch debriefing discussions. Although we have taken measures to protect the anonymity of the aftercare facilities, the descriptions below are of actual historical entities which have already evolved during the intervening years.

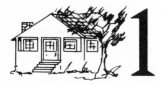 1 # THE STUDY

INTRODUCTION

In this book the experiences of suicidal patients who have been treated in a mental hospital and have been discharged into residential aftercare facilities are explored. Many previous studies have examined the pre- and inhospital feelings and reactions of suicidal psychiatric patients, but very little has been published on the crucial period immediately following departure from the hospital. One of our own studies, *Suicide: Inside and Out* (1976), focused on suicide within the hospital. This volume is a natural sequel, covering the first few weeks after discharge and applying the same method of experiential research to the study of suicide within several kinds of residential aftercare facilities.

The primary reason for conducting these studies has been to seek answers to the question: How can we improve the help we offer to persons who have undergone emotional distress so painful that it has brought them to the point either of contemplating self-destruction or of actually attempting it? We have learned from previous work that such a point is neither lightly nor quickly reached. Instead, it is more likely to be the end point of a long series of events stretching over a number of years, events that have brought deep despair for person and family and have led to close contacts with clergymen, physicians, agencies, and mental health professionals, and perhaps even to sojourns in medical and/or mental hospitals. When these various sources of help do not succeed in resolving the conflicts, the final "solution" of self-termination has been contemplated or experienced.

The neuropsychiatric hospital is for many suicidal patients a last resort, used when self-control has dissipated, judgment has disappeared, and a structured environment is needed, at least to reconstitute if not to cure. For most of its patients the hospital does provide significant help; for a small number it does not. The percentage of patients who kill themselves each year in the Veterans Administration's large system of neuropsychiatric hospitals is infinitesimal, about .00025 (Farberow et al., 1971). The small size of this figure, however, does not obscure the fact that practically all suicides are premature, unhappy, and generally unnecessary. An important fact about neuropsychiatric hospital suicides has emerged in repeated studies. By far the majority of the deaths, between two-thirds and three-fourths, occurred after the patients left the hospital, usually within a few months. What happened to the patients during these weeks to make them once more feel suicidal? What made them lose hope? What prompted them to act out their feelings of despair, or anger, or guilt, rather than returning to the hospital for available help? What were their thoughts, their feelings, their moods? What contacts, interactions, and relationships with people restimulated pain so intense that the prospect of having to adjust once again within the community became unbearable? "Certified" as well enough to leave the hospital and having progressed thus far, why do they kill themselves at this stage? Using experiential research as the investigative procedure, we designed this study to answer the above questions.

EXPERIENTIAL RESEARCH

Our reasons for using experiential research techniques have been outlined in detail in *Suicide: Inside and Out.* The reader is referred to that volume for a complete description of the process, with its pros and cons, and for discussion of the experiences of other researchers in the use of this method. For the reader's convenience, however, a brief summary of the important points is given here.

In the past, researchers in this field have had to rely on the suicidal patient's own recollections and comments to gain insight into his hospital experiences and into his relationships with others. In most instances, his reconstruction of his experiences, usually developed after the event, was colored by the selective process of his memory. Experiential research, however, emplaces a trained observer who can report on his own subjective experiences and on the events that happen around him. Prior training and experience help him to delineate these internal and external events critically. The researcher is his own expert informant.

This method has been used before, primarily in mental hospitals, where the social realities of the ward and its staff and the individual realities of the patients are in continuous interaction. The researcher continually keeps in mind two questions of equal importance: "What is going on within me?" and "What is going on in the setting around me?" The researcher introspects, observes, and participates in a complex interplay of sensory, perceptual, and cognitive experience.

Anthropological studies have traditionally used the participation-observation technique, which requires the researcher to live among the people he is studying with the aim of getting at their understanding of their world. Experiential research differs significantly from this technique. In the traditional method the focus is on other persons. What is happening within the researcher is either disregarded or given little weight, although it is acknowledged that the anthropologist affects the people he is observing and the data he is gathering. In experiential research that investigator does not create a new role; rather he adopts one that is already operational within the system in which he chooses to live.

The main methodological problem of experiential research is that of replication and generalization. The researcher's observations are personal accounts based on a changing instrument operating in an evolving social setting. It is possible, however, to generate supplemental information which can be used in evaluations. The refinement we have used in our experiential research is the introduction of a second researcher, Helen Summers, into the same setting at the same time. David Kent and Helen Summers are identities we created and activated. They are alike in many ways, primarily in their histories of depression and suicide attempts. By placing them simultaneously into the same setting we hoped to discover which elements of David Kent's responses to his environment resulted from his unique perception and which stemmed from situational pressures on a particular class of persons (suicidal, depressive, ex-patients who are stigmatized outcasts). To be sure, other comparisons in these and other settings were required, but we saw the use of a second researcher as a first step in "calibrating" our "instrument."

Another way to forestall bias is to have the researcher list his expectations before entering the setting so that they can later be checked against his actual experiences. If expectations and experiences differ markedly, the research is more likely to be valid.

In experiential research the investigator has to commit a great deal of time to the project. First he has to prepare his new identity and then he has to remain in the experiential setting for a period long enough to enable him to accumulate a worthwhile store of information. At times there may even be potential danger, physical and psychological.

The ethical problem is one that probably will never be completely resolved. Some investigators believe that any kind of deception in research is to be avoided at all costs. Our feeling, however, is that the means and the ends in any project must be carefully evaluated: Will the results justify the personal investments in and the subjective costs of the research? In this study, peer residents and staff did not know the true identity of the searcher-patient or researcher-resident. The owners and managers of the agencies, however, did know that a researcher would be living in their facilities for an unspecified period during some previously arranged broad span of time. We made every effort to diminish their feeling of being deceived by obtaining permission from the aftercare facility owners beforehand and by contacting staff and fellow residents afterward. The goals of the project were explained thoroughly, both before and after the live-in experience. In each setting, after the experiential phase of the research had been completed, we asked staff members for their reactions to our experiential observations and used their responses to supplement our own findings. We offered suggestions for changes which we felt would improve the setting for all role groups. A noncritical, nonthreatening personal posture was adopted throughout. The reader can judge for himself the advantages and disadvantages of this method as he reads the day-by-day account of the researcher's experiences and the reports of the debriefings held with staff members afterward.

One other feature of the method of experiential research is inherent in the process and in the kinds of observations obtained. In the earlier experience in a psychiatric ward, we found that David Kent, the researcher-patient, and his fellow patients were responding in common human ways to the situational pressures exerted on them. Despite all kinds of differences in background — genetic structure, childhood experiences, and cultural absorption — the common humanity of each person emerged.

Scales, questionnaires, projective tests, and other techniques aim for surface or in-depth measurements of personality traits, attitude complexes, and behavior styles. Continuity is presumed to exist within the individual; to confirm that continuity, psychologists give the same tests later on to the same person. We feel, however, that the continuity lies not in the person per se, but in situated persons. Situations provide continuity of response from persons who actually have multiple and flexible personality traits, that is, numerous identities. In other words, in order to understand behavior we must know as much about the setting as we do about the person. Taking our conception a step further, we feel that an individual's replies in written tests (fixed-choice or open-ended questions) are not necessarily projections of his responses to situations other than the one in which the tests were first given. Much research in the field of depression and suicide requires people to take tests of various sorts in situations of various sorts. The key idea is that repeated behaviors by a person over a period of time are not necessarily the product of an underlying or pervasive personality trait, but that they may rather be a function of common aspects of the situations in which the individual finds himself. It may be simpler — but it may also be incorrect — to assume that he behaves consistently because of his personality organization and not because of consistencies in settings.

THE SETTING

Broadly speaking, three possible settings confront a neuropsychiatric hospital patient immediately after discharge: he may live alone; he may live with his family; he may live in a residential aftercare facility. Our study focuses on the latter. In principle, aftercare facilities are used as residences for discharged mental hospital patients because they provide continuity of care. The patient who leaves the hospital has been in a highly structured, well-regulated, and tightly organized institution. Since the responsibility for his life there has been assumed by others, all he must do is focus on recovery from his emotional distress. The transition from so controlled an environment to a community where he must assume, or resume, full responsibility for his conduct has often proven too abrupt and stressful. Some aftercare facilities are designed to serve as a bridge back to the community; they provide relatively less structured care and emphasize a gradual increase in the patient's control over his own activities and interests. Other aftercare facilities become permanent residences for those who will never be able to adjust to the outside world.

Residential aftercare facilities vary in size and condition and philosophy of management. At the time of our research, the smallest ones were called family-care units. In an ordinary single-family house the ex-patient lives with the manager and from one to five other residents. Many of these family-care units are run "family style," with the household members eating together, taking trips together, and so forth. The atmosphere of such a place depends largely on the interest and the life style of the manager. Larger facilities, housing up to about 150 residents, are called board-and-care facilities. Occupying large houses or apartmentlike structures, they provide room and board and varying degrees of supervision, recreation, and rehabilitation.

A survey (Chase, Gross, Hanna, Israel, and Woods, 1970) of fifteen board-and-care homes utilized by a Los Angeles Veterans Administration (VA) psychiatric hospital produced the following descriptive profile. A resident shares his bedroom with one person and his bathroom with four others. The apartment house is usually in a residential area near a laundry, a grocery and liquor store, a coffee shop, and a bus stop. The management provides a television viewing room and other recreational facilities, such as Ping-Pong, checkers, chess and sometimes a pool. Staff members prepare and serve meals and distribute medications. Most of the residents are middle-aged males. The survey describes eight of the homes as "impersonal" and seven as "homey." Ten evoked a warm, lively mood; five were sterile and coldly institutional. Two had bad odors and two were dirty. Only three of the facilities included residents who were not mentally disturbed.

The sponsors (owners and/or managers) of these facilities tended to come from related occupations: nine had operated rest homes before and two had been nurses. Only two owners had had no experience with psychiatric patients before opening their facilities. They gave as the main reason for selecting this occupation an interest in people; second was the desire to make a profit. Nevertheless, there were disadvantages: heavy demands on their time, frequent emotional strain, trouble finding and keeping staff, licensing problems, and low financial returns on their investments. When asked the purpose of the facility, nine of the fifteen sponsors said they hoped "to get the person out on his own into the community"; five acknowledged a desire "to provide a good home and a family atmosphere"; and one straightforwardly wanted "to run a good business."

The opposing themes of "stepping-stones into the community" and "warehouses for people" appeared often in the sponsors' accounts. Confusion in their minds about the purpose of residential aftercare facilities is reflected in their uncertainity as to the best methods of operating such institutions. Chase et al. (1970) point out that maintenance-oriented homes prodded their residents into seeking out activities in the community, whereas rehabilitation-oriented homes encouraged activities on the premises, as mental hospitals do. In other words, some residents who were supposedly in training for community reentry were deprived of community experience by the training itself.

In sum, residential aftercare facilities are life settings of various sizes and of differing quality for former psychiatric patients who do not return to families or to independent living. They may serve as a traditional bridge between the hospital and independent community living, or they may more or less permanently house people who do not need hospitalization but who are unable to function self-sufficiently in the larger society. Frequently, a single facility fulfills both functions: some residents stay and some go out on their own. Sometimes residents must return to the hospital.

PREPARATION

The techniques we used to develop suicidal identities in experimental researchers are described in detail in *Suicide: Inside and Out* (Reynolds and Farberow, 1976). Essentially, they involved role playing with professional feedback. Slumped posture, sighs and shallow breathing, slow movements, and repetitious internal messages of hopelessness supported the newly depressed, recently suicidal "self." The same identity used for David Kent (DKR) in the hospital was continued in the aftercare facilities. Briefly, his identity was that of a shy, withdrawn, introspective, self-doubting young man. He had a protective mother and a father who had left home when David was six. He also had a sister, a year and a half younger than he. When Kent was discharged from the navy he went to Saint Petersburg, Florida, where his mother was living. He entered college but dropped out shortly afterward when his mother died. He was hard hit by his mother's death. After a few years of working at odd jobs he met and married his wife. He felt that she was wonderful, but troubles loomed when he lost his job and could not find another. She finally left him, and a series of reconciliations and separations followed.

Kent came to California on the promise of a job in the aerospace industry, but nothing materialized, and other efforts to find work were unsuccessful. When he called his wife on their wedding anniversary she told him she wanted a divorce; she would not come out to California, as had been planned. David thereupon made a suicide attempt with Seconal, but he was found and was taken to the General Hospital Emergency Receiving Unit. After his stomach was pumped out, he was discharged. When two days later he was found wandering the streets, he was taken to a VA hospital. He spent two weeks there and then was discharged. The account of his experiences in the hospital is reported in *Suicide: Inside and Out.*

Because DKR had so thoroughly immersed himself in his David Kent identity, it was unnecessary to rebuild that identity in preparation for his entry into the aftercare setting. Indeed, while waiting for the social worker who would accompany him to the board-and-care home, simply sitting in the dayroom of a ward like the one in which he had earlier been hospitalized helped change David Reynolds back into David Kent. Perhaps the most powerful influences, however, came only after the researchers were in the actual setting and were perceived to be depressed ex-patients by those in their new social world. It was difficult to resist the force of others' expectations, expressed in both subtle and obvious messages.

As indicated earlier, we expanded our methodology for the present study by using a second researcher placed in a board-and-care home at the same time for the same length of time. At the time of the study Helen Summers was a graduate student in psychology serving an internship in the psychology department of a VA neuropsychiatric hospital. She had had previous experience working in a board-and-care home in Boston. A suicidal identity was developed for her also. Preparation, however, was not so intense as it had been for David Kent, for in an aftercare home she would not be subjected to as much observation as in the hospital.

Helen's background story, like David Kent's, was a blend of experienced reality and imaginative creation. Helen Summers, aged twenty-four, was born in Springfield, Massachusetts, the eldest of three daughters. When she was very young the family moved to a small town in Connecticut. There she spent the rest of her childhood, graduating from high school in 1966. She attended a little-known junior college near Boston and then stayed in the city another year to work as a laboratory assistant in a university. Because she was undecided about what to do with her life, she enlisted in the navy. For three years, stationed at New London, Connecticut, she worked as a laboratory technician.

During this period Helen met Lew, a journalist working on the base newspaper. After two years of courtship they planned to marry in June despite the objection of Helen's parents. Both Helen and Lew were discharged in May, but then Lew decided that he did not want to be tied down by marriage after all. Instead, he wanted to go back to an Indian reservation where he had once lived and to spend his time there writing. By the last-minute change in plans Lew thus confirmed the accusations of unreliability made by Helen's parents. Helen, who had made plans only for the wedding, felt she could not tell her parents of her sudden loss of a predictable future. She became depressed. Staying with friends in Cambridge, Massachusetts, solved no problems; it merely postponed their solution. Troubled by insomnia, she started to take sleeping pills. Finally, she decided that a complete change and a new start were necessary. In June she spent most of her savings on a bus ticket to Los Angeles. Arriving there, she was awed by the strangeness of the city. She had no friends, no one to talk with, no job. After two weeks, with her money dwindling, she took an overdose of sleeping pills. The motel manager found her and took her to a local hospital. She was transferred to a VA hospital, treated, and discharged to B Home.

APPROACHING THE SPONSORS

A number of sponsors from residential aftercare facilities were approached with our research proposal. They were told of our earlier experience in a VA hospital. The risks of the study and the potential benefits to them, to suicidal persons in particular, and to psychiatric patients in general were carefully explained. The sponsors were invited to sign up for the program if they were willing to accept an unidentified researcher as a resident for an unspecified period of time in the role of a former psychiatric hospital patient. In return, the researchers agreed to discuss their observations with facility staff members during postresearch debriefing sessions and with the group of sponsors as a whole when the entire project was completed. Volunteering to participate was no guarantee that any particular facility would be selected, since we did not know at that point how many settings we could enter in the six months projected for the live-in phase of the project.

In all, five board-and-care homes and five family-care units agreed to participate in our research. Of these, we were able to study four residences with designated capacities of three, fifteen, twenty-three, and ninety residents — a good spread in terms of size. The neighborhoods represented, including a low-income black area, a low-income racially mixed area, and a middle-income white area, again provided a reasonably wide range.

Our previous experience in placing David Kent in a VA hospital had alerted us to most of the potential difficulties in establishing an acceptable, documented identity, so that arranging placement in the aftercare residences without arousing suspicion proved to be relatively easy, especially with the assistance of cooperating social workers. A social service summary report was prepared (see Appendix). A two-week hospitalization history was created; names of ward personnel were memorized. Kent was given a daily work assignment at the hospital when he was placed in two nearby settings. Social workers supplied information about the clothing and personal items that would be appropriate to take to the residences. It was decided to prescribe genuine antidepressant medication for the researchers, but they were to avoid taking it, if possible. Our NIMH grant provided funds for the usual room and board in each residence (at that time $198 a month). Each researcher carried twenty dollars in pocket money.

Each placement was made in the customary way by a VA social worker who made a phone call from the hospital to the aftercare facility. Arrangements for transfer were completed at that time.

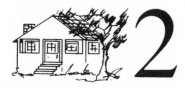

2 COMMUNITY CARE: AN OVERVIEW

Background

Community treatment of discharged neuropsychiatric patients has a long history. The tradition of caring for the mentally ill in family settings originated in Geel, near Antwerp, Belgium, in the sixth century A.D., when an Irish princess, Dymphna, fled from her home because her insane father had incestuous designs on her. She was overtaken in Geel and decapitated. The people in the community enshrined both the place of her death and her remains, and the Catholic church encouraged the belief that her shrine had healing properties for the insane.

Today the people of Geel continue to care for mentally ill patients by placing them with local families. Having learned that mental patients are rarely dangerous, they have continued to participate in this community rehabilitation program for hundreds of years. Dumont and Aldrich (1962) compare fifty-six Geel families that continued to accept patients with forty-seven families that had accepted mental patients in the past but no longer did so. Their findings reveal that families in the former category appeared to be more closely knit and that they were often headed by farmers or white-collar workers of modest income. Families that had dropped out of the program were usually headed by professionals or entrepreneurs with a slightly higher level of income.

Norway's long history of treating mental patients outside the hospital or asylum dates back to the tenth century. Only within the past twenty years, however, has there been a significant increase in the proportion of mentally ill persons lodged in extramural care

11

facilities, largely because Norwegian hospitals are overcrowded and because community care costs about a third or a fourth as much as hospital care. According to David (1962), who surveyed the entire hospital system in Norway, more psychiatric patients are now being cared for in homes, private facilities, or nursing homes than in hospitals.

In Scotland, the boarding out of patients was considered highly desirable. The Scots believe that in this way the mentally ill would become accustomed to a sane society and could more easily be educated and trained to function in society once more and to reestablish a normal pattern of living. Massachusetts started its foster-home program in 1885. By 1970 twenty-two other states had established similar systems. The VA initiated its program in 1951 and is now probably the chief proponent of foster-home care in the United States. In twenty-three years more than 7,500 veteran patients accumulated more than 38,000 placements in foster homes.

The major trend in community psychiatry during the past two decades has been toward early release of hospital patients back to the community, along with outpatient support. The objective is to prevent frequent returns to the hospital and to circumvent chronicity. Some observers have even predicted the demise of the mental institutions, as community mental health centers were established and the use of board-and-care homes and foster homes continued to increase. Lamb and Goertzel (1971, 1972), for example, note the large numbers of patients discharged from Agnew State Hospital in California. Consistent with nationwide trends, the total Agnew patient population was reduced from 3,666 to 986 during a five-year follow-up period, a decline of 73 percent. Lamb and Goertzel also found that approximately 20 percent of the sample, particularly assaultive patients and those who presented management problems that private facilities could not handle, continued to require services that only the hospital could provide. Fifty percent of the ex-patients living in the community were at least partly self-supporting, but many of them were more isolated and withdrawn than they had been in the hospital. After five years very few patients had become completely self-supporting; most remained marginal and inadequate. Many of the boarding houses were privately owned and profit-oriented. The operators did not want to invest in additional staff for vocational rehabilitation, even though vocational and rehabilitation-oriented living facilities were the most successful. The latter included professionally run satellite apartment programs, halfway houses, and other transitional housing arrangements. Patients living in noninstitutional settings (alone, with family or relative, or in satellite housing) functioned at a higher vocational level than patients in boarding houses. Placement of patients in foster homes was seen as an obvious step in helping the hospital achieve its goal of preparing patients to function adequately in the community. In addition, sending a patient back to his own family when it continued to breed pathology or failed to offer support was deemed unwise.

Morrissey (1965) reviews the movement toward family care (a term used, for the most part, synonymously with foster-home care) for mental patients and assesses the resistance shown by some states to participation in that program. The reasons for their reluctance are the difficulty in finding suitable homes, in identifying reliable criteria for the selection of appropriate patients, and in optimally matching patients to sponsors; legal problems in launching a family-care program; staff shortages; the American tradition of rugged individualism; and organized resistance stemming from fears within the community. Studies relevant to the selection of patients for family care, Morrissey concludes, are badly needed.

Prediction of Success

Does community placement work? Is the use of foster-home care and community treatment generally successful? Research on foster care has focused almost exclusively on patient characteristics; it has been conducted in terms of success or failure in staying out of the hospital and in maintaining community tenure. Questions have been raised as to whether "staying out" is the best criterion of success, or whether it is preferable to inpatient care for many individuals. Nothing was known about the patient's personal comfort and adjustment in foster homes as compared with the alternative of continuing hospitalization. Friedman, von Mering, and Hinko (1966) suggest that the chronic schizophrenic is always with us and that what has been created is the condition of "intermittent patienthood." They point out that, in the rush to put people into the community, little more has been accomplished than to create a different type of institution housing sheltered subsocieties, which then serve as a base for periodic return to the hospital for treatment. In a follow-up study covering five to six years in the lives of 1,037 patients admitted to a short-term treatment hospital in Cleveland in one calendar year, Friedman and his colleagues found that approximately 64 percent were rehospitalized. The authors also feel that the high release rate reflected in part the introduction and widespread use of psychotropic drugs.

On the other side of the issue, Lamb and associates (1967) are highly critical of those who have opposed community treatment of mentally ill patients. Their guiding principle is that community treatment should be primary, since continued hospitalization fosters dependency, regression, apathy, and alienation from family and community. The problem, however, is to make sure that community facilities are directed toward improvement and not simply toward maintenance. Isolation from the mainstream of society in certain board-and-care homes can be as limiting as existence in some state hospitals. The authors feel that, while the number of patients transferred from hospital to community has sharply increased, too little attention has been paid to rehabilitation in the community care facilities.

In a follow-up study of "high-expectation" placement (a halfway house experience followed by satellite housing and day treatment centers or rehabilitation workshops) versus "low-expectation" placement (board-and-care and family-care homes) for long-term state mental hospital patients, Lamb and Goertzel (1971) found that members of the high-expectation group made much more progress. They were less segregated from the general community and, despite a higher rehospitalization rate, were able to stay out of the hospital longer than those in the low-expectation group. Lamb and his associates (1967) list the following criteria for treatment of the long-term patient in a community care facility. (1) The patient must receive close attention at the time of his first psychotic episode. (2) High but realistic expectations must be maintained so that the patient strives to realize his full social and vocational potential, even though the potential may be limited. (3) Efforts must be directed to giving the patient a sense of mastery, a feeling that he can cope with his drives, his symptoms, and his environment. (4) The more care a facility gives the patient, the higher the degree of envelopment; the optimal degree of envelopment is what is needed to make the patient's living situation as noninstitutional as possible. (5) Goals must be clearly defined for each long-term patient, especially limited goals that can be accomplished in the time available; sheltered workshops and individual psychotherapy are helpful. (6) Work therapy should be a cornerstone of community treatment of the long-term patient. (7) The mental patient needs to learn, and should be permitted to regain, the status of "normal community resident." (8) Normalization of the patient's environment must always be the goal.

A number of studies have attempted to isolate specific factors that would predict success in community care of mentally ill persons. Ullmann, Berkman, and Hamister (1958) used psychological material as a basis for predictions in regard to VA hospital patients. The results of such tests as the Rorschach, TAT, Porteus Mazes, MMPI, and Sentence Completion were compared with ratings of patient conformity after placement, the number of years of NP hospitalization before placement, and percentage gain scores, that is, the percentage of time the patient stayed out of the hospital in the period from his first placement to the cutoff date of the study. The psychological test results showed an insignificant relationship to length of stay in the community. The investigators found that the length of prior NP hospitalization was the best criterion for predicting how long the patient would remain outside the hospital, with a positive correlation of 0.65 between the length of prior NP hospitalization and a posthospital adjustment scale. They also discovered that personality evaluation reports written by ward social workers when the patient was referred to a home-care facility were less significant as predictors of outcome than were the length of NP hospitalization and the type of ward patient (more or less regressed).

In a later study, Ullmann and Berkman (1959a) used the criterion of time subsequently spent in an NP hospital to contrast the efficacy of family care versus hospitalization for VA neuropsychiatric patients. Using a minimum follow-up period of eighteen months and a sample of 191 VA hospital patients placed in family-care homes for trial visits, the investigators found that 33 percent were readmitted to the hospital, 29 percent were still living in the home-care facilities, and 38 percent were living independently. Thus by the end of the follow-up period 67 percent of the patients had not had to return to the hospital. The median proportion of time spent out of psychiatric hospitals from first hospitalization to first placement was 25 percent, as contrasted with 90.5 percent from first placement to the study's follow-up date. The authors conclude that, for their sample, a median of an additional six months of every year was spent out of psychiatric hospitals after home-care placement.

Lyle and Trail (1961) studied, over a three-year period, sixty-nine patients placed in foster homes by a VA hospital in the state of Washington. Their findings revealed that forty-six patients remained out of the hospital continuously for more than two years after placement and that twenty-three "nonadjusted" patients required readmission to the hospital within two years because of suicidal problems or failure to maintain psychiatric stability. Patients who seemed to fit best in the foster homes were characterized by predictability or stability of their behavior within the hospital, capacity for relating to other people in their environment (social interaction with other patients, staff, etc.), and lack of initiative or drive toward changing their situation. These qualities tended to be associated with patients over forty years of age and with those who had been hospitalized for periods of more than ten years. Lyle and Trail conclude that patients who conformed most closely to the behavior expectations of the hospital staff were most likely to adjust to home-care placement. A favorable attitude toward leaving the hospital was negatively related to home-care adjustment. About 91 percent of the nonadjusted group, versus 57 percent of the adjusted group, wanted to leave the hospital.

A study of forty-three patients from three VA neuropsychiatric hospitals (Linn, Brown, Miller, Thompson, and Wathan, 1966) evaluated the patients on an adjustment rating scale and then classified them in good, fair, and poor adjustment groups. This study corroborates previous findings that past hospital experience was the most significant factor in the ability to adjust: three or more previous hospitalizations related to poor adjustment, whereas total number of years (10 to 20) in the hospital related to good adjustment. The most suitable candidates for placement were chronic patients with histories of long single hospitalization, though older patients were less likely to make good adjustments. Black patients were found to adjust relatively better to family care; poor adjustment was related to having lived alone prior to hospitalization. Patients who made better adjustments had had more visits from relatives while they were hospitalized. Perhaps oddly, patients who were most optimistic in their attitude toward placement tended to make the poorest adjustment. Foster families in rural environments with a relatively high tolerance for deviant behavior tended to have patients who made good adjustments. Patients placed in families of the same religious faith as their own made better adjustments.

Cunningham, Botwinik, Dolson, and Weickert (1969) conducted a five-year study of 111 patients drawn from a VA hospital and placed in community homes. The forty-four who remained in the community two years or longer were considered "successful"; the sixty-seven who returned to the hospital within twenty-four months were considered not successful. Twenty-eight percent of the return-ees went back to the hospital within the first month of placement, the most critical period. Eighty-one percent of those who returned to the hospital did so within a year of placement.

This study also found that the longer the period of prior NP hospitalization, the higher were the patient's chances of remaining in the community for a longer period of time. Patients who were active in the community — holding jobs and attending day center rehabilita-tion programs — also tended to remain in the community longer. Younger patients were more successful in community homes than older patients. The larger the size of the community home, the longer the patient was likely to remain in the community. Widowed, single, and married patients tended to stay in the community longer than separated or divorced patients. Patients with longer periods of military service also tended to remain in the community longer.

Factor analysis was used by McCarthy, Alkire, and Pearman (1965) to identify sets of related variables which could predict success or failure in home-care placement of mental patients from a VA hospital. The most common variables were found to be interper-sonal conflict within the home, covert aggression or hostility, overt aggression or hostility, predictability of behavior (sponsor's satisfac-tion with patient), use of alcohol, and physical health.

In a later study, Alkire, Pearman, and McCarthy (1966) com-pared the backgrounds and attitudes of NP patients (veterans) placed in home care with the backgrounds and attitudes of the sponsors of the homes in which the patients were placed. The outcome of placement was felt to be a function of the compatibility of a particular patient with a particular sponsor. The authors found that the most important factors in predicting conflict between patient and sponsor were alcohol abuse, including alcohol use by the parents of the patient, and past trouble between the patient and the police.

Lee (1963) studied over a thirty-month period the characteristics of mental patients selected from a state hospital for family-care placement and determined the factors for prediction of success. The critical period, he reports, was the first eighty-nine days of placement, when 19 percent of all patients placed in family care returned to the hospital. The patients who were most successful in remaining in family care homes for a longer period of time were those who had had a longer NP hospitalization before placement.

Lorei and Gurel (1972) analyzed a 91-item true/false inventory of the patient's history and state of well-being used to predict posthospital employment and readmission of 720 male schizophrenics placed in the community after treatment in a VA hospital. The instruments were the 77-item Palo Alto Social Background Inventory and 14 items from a work-study scale. In the nine-month period following the patients' release from the hospital, the researchers found, 50 percent of the sample did not work at all and 33 percent were readmitted to the hospital. The major findings were that work success depended upon (in decreasing order of importance) chronicity of hospitalization, total recent earnings, patients' perception of their own disability (those viewing themselves as least disabled enjoyed the greatest success), marital status, and uncritical optimism. The authors did not find that scale scores were related to hospital readmission.

Gurel and Lorei later (1972) used a symptom rating scale to measure psychopathology in 951 male schizophrenics under sixty years of age just prior to hospital release. They then obtained the same scale ratings three months and nine months after release. Not all the patients in the sample went into community care facilities, but the results are significant in terms of employment and readmission. Gurel and Lorei found little relationship between ratings of symptoms of psychopathology and subsequent readmission to the hospital. Employment was much more predictable than readmission to the hospital. Low motivation was the major factor in work failure; contributing factors were anticipation of restricted psychosocial functioning, depression, slovenly appearance, and cognitive impairment. In other words, psychopathology and related symptoms were clearly related to success in finding and holding employment. Gurel and Lorei (1972) concluded, however, that psychiatric hospitals were minimally effective in preparing patients for continued community membership and productive employment.

Carhill (1968) describes the community care program for California's state mental hospital patients as primarily directed toward placement of elderly, chronically ill, indigent patients. The shift of 1,577 patients over a period of two and a half years contributed markedly to reducing the population of California mental hospitals, but no report on the benefits derived by the patients from their community care living was available.

Kemp (1972) interviewed approximately 160 former patients of a VA mental hospital in Los Angeles who participated in a program that included outpatient contact after discharge. If rehospitalization was necessary, the patient returned to the same ward and thus received continuous support from a staff familiar to him. Kemp found that half the patients lived in board-and-care facilities, about 16 percent lived alone or with friends, 18 percent with their wives; and 11 percent with parents or relatives. Those patients who returned to a marriage situation functioned at a higher level than the others. Work history was spotty: 37 percent never worked a full year at any one job; most of the patients found sporadic short-term employment. In general, Kemp found that the patients continued to be dependent on the hospital and to hold onto their relationship with it. Many of them, in fact, did not consider themselves discharged; they felt that they were still in the hospital even though they were living on the outside.

Linn, Caffey, Klett, and Hogarty (1975) studied the value and effectiveness of preparation for and placement in foster care. They assigned 572 subjects from five hospitals randomly to foster-care preparation or to continued hospitalization. They studied the patients before assignment to foster-care facilities, at the time of placement, and four months later. The hospitals averaged about two months in preparing the patients for foster care and were able to place 73 percent. Patients were measured with a 21-item Social Dysfunction Rating Scale, the Katz Adjustment Rating Scale, and the Clyde Mood Scale, along with ratings on the Discharge Readiness Inventory.

The major findings were that patients showed little or no change in social functioning, mood, activity, and adjustment as the result of hospital preparation for foster care. Within four months after going into foster-care homes, however, experimental subjects showed significant improvement over controlled subjects, particularly in ability to function and in overall adjustment. Whether short or long preparation for placement was given, no difference in relapse rates or in the number of days the patients stayed in foster care, was evident. The major changes in adjustment occurred after foster-care placement. Although mood probably interacted with other variables in producing differences in overall change, mood in itself did not show significant variation. Likewise, activity levels, though expected to change under foster care, failed to differentiate experimentals from controls at either placement or follow-up.

Chase, Gross, Hanna, Israel, and Woods (1970) investigated the physical and structural characteristics, as well as the orientation, of fifteen board-and-care homes housing ten or more mental patients released from the VA neuropsychiatric hospital in Los Angeles. They found that almost all the homes were maintenance-oriented, with only one of the fifteen actively encouraging patients to move on to independent living. Many of the establishments, however, did encourage patients to seek activities outside the home. The one home that was rehabilitation-oriented resembled the hospital in providing all activities on the premises.

There was an obvious lack of work-oriented activities for patients in these board-and-care homes. The omission is a significant failing, for the ability of ex-patients to find employment is severely limited, owing to the stigma of mental illness. The homes were found to be primarily apartment-type buildings housing a middle-aged population; the investigators discerned a definite need for more resources for young Vietnam war veterans. Some patients seemed to be better suited to a maintenance home while others would have profited more from a rehabilitative program. What was most needed was a more effective placement method to ensure the best match of patient to home.

The consistent findings in all research projects relating to mental hospitals and aftercare facilities thus demonstrate the superiority of foster care, and the relatively low relapse rates confirm its usefulness, not only as a family substitute but also as a stepping-stone to a wider community life. Most of the studies show that treatment in community care establishments has been both successful and desirable for most mental hospital patients. The first weeks after discharge seem to be the critical period for all patients, whether or not they are suicidal. Why are these first weeks so critical in leading either to rehospitalization, as these studies show, or to suicide, as our statistical data indicate? Why is the fit between sponsor and resident a crucial factor in an ex-patient's adjustment to life outside the hospital? Our research makes a start in providing detailed answers to these questions. Aftercare facilities are small societies in themselves, and this volume offers insight into the social life in these oases of human interaction. The journal accounts that follow form the heart of this book. They describe the actual experiences of the experimental researchers who lived in the aftercare residences.

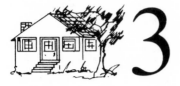

B HOME

The first facility to be described, which we call B Home, is the largest of the four that were used in the study. The two researchers, David Kent and Helen Summers, entered this facility at the same time. B Home comprises several units, the largest of which is an apartment-like structure housing nearly a hundred patients. The social worker described it as follows: "B Home has a staff of approximately fifteen. There is a good deal of structure, including programs in the areas of recreation and occupational therapy. The sponsors are genuinely interested in and concerned with the residents in their charge. Their focus, however, is on the resident being made 'happy' and remaining in the home. The size and scope of the facility give it the atmosphere of a small hospital, so dependency may be fostered. Privacy is limited, with four to five residents assigned to a single sleeping area. The home can be used for veterans needing a custodial-type placement. Medication and funds are closely supervised. Public transportation is convenient and the home provides bus service to the hospital for those who cannot travel by themselves."

The following account is an edited journal of Kent's experiences in B Home.

KENT'S B HOME JOURNAL

August 7

At 2:30 P.M. I was waiting with the social worker for the bus from B Home to pick me up. If a patient is ambivalent or has fears about leaving, his social worker may take him to visit the aftercare facility before placing him there, but I went in "cold," without knowing much about the place and without having first visited it.

The bus driver greeted me with natural friendliness. The first-name basis of acquaintanceship was set up at once. It was Leon and Don and Karl and David right from the start. During the bus ride, with its masculine atmosphere, the talk was about cars and women. A pleasant camaraderie prevailed.

A resident helped me carry my luggage inside. We left my suitcase and cardboard box by the pool while I went upstairs to sign in. Several people had already greeted me. A lady in the office filled in some forms, and I signed a card. The bus driver showed me the TV room and dining hall and then took me to my room. I was instructed to keep my key with me all the time because the outside doors are locked at night. The hours for eating and for riding the bus were also explained, just once. In the newness of my situation, names and instructions weren't filtering through very well, but there was written and verbal repetition to the extent needed. Lack of instructions about details of living (such as whether towels are provided and when linen is changed) forced me to watch others to see what they did and to ask questions. Both activities effectively draw out the resident who wishes to fit into the routine. The structuring of social systems to provide natural opportunities for cooperative interaction needs theoretical and practical research.

The sheets on my bed were unchanged, the light bulb was burned out, and the closet door had left its track. The driver noticed the door and told me it would be fixed promptly, as it was. Karl, a handyman, came in and fixed it as I was putting my clothes away.

Karl was the middle-level person who held the community together. Every institution has such a person (Reynolds, 1976). He knew what was happening around the facility, knew the patients by name, worked and played alongside management and patients, and generally was a focus of community activity. His friendly, open manner was nicely balanced by an active work orientation. Such a person is useful in that he avoids the artificiality of "therapizing"; the lessons he teaches and the model he offers are translatable into the patient's daily life simply because he is a co-worker, a participant in the patient's world.

I worried more about homosexual advances in this setting than in the hospital. There was less supervision and protection, more freedom and privacy. There had as yet been no overt moves, so my

concern was diminishing. There were several self-proclaimed homo-
sexuals but they didn't seem to bother the others.

The physical layout of my room was therapeutic for the withdrawn, suicidal resident. I was given some privacy but it was difficult
to be alone. Six residents shared a bathroom and there was a natural
traffic flow through the space in which I lived. As a result, there were
natural opportunities for interaction without people looking in,
prying, or otherwise artificially stimulating social contact.

After putting my things away I went outside and sat on a chair
by the pool. Another patient started a conversation.

"Hi! My name is Albert."

"My name is David."

"David?"

(I nod.)

"Glad to meet you."

"Glad to meet you."

"Where're you from?"

"Ohio, originally."

"From the Veterans [Hospital] ?"

"Yes."

"That's fine."

My name and where I am from (not where I was born or where I
had lived, but what hospital and what psychiatric ward I came from)
are the data sought in greeting. Just as in parts of the rural South one
"counts kin" when meeting a stranger to find a common relative, or
as at a cocktail party one asks a person's profession, we all need
information that will enable us to relate to strangers. Finding a
hospital or a particular ward in common helps to define a newcomer's relationships.

My roommate was black. He was quiet but seemed willing to be
helpful. One resident in the room between mine and the front door
spent a lot of time lying on his bed. He mumbled and hallucinated
but was very clean and friendly. Said he was Clark Gable's son. (We
also had an ex-girl friend of Bob Hope's.)

I took a 20-minute nap, and at 5:00 P.M. I went to supper.
Earlier it had been announced over the loudspeaker that there would
be a residents' meeting just before we ate. The purpose was to
introduce new houseparents and new residents and to ask how many
of us wanted to go to the Dodgers' ball game. The meeting lasted five
minutes. Medication in individual envelopes was passed out to us at
suppertime. It was easy to slip the pills into my pocket.

After supper I sat, wrote notes in my room, lay down, read, and wandered around. Already I had acquired a feel for the characteristic social groupings in this facility. There were several areas for socializing — a line of chairs under a balcony, poolside chairs, lobby chairs, an area in front of B Home where people gathered, the TV room, the canteen, and chairs by the phone. There was both mixed and segregated interaction by sex and by race (blacks, Mexican Americans, and whites). Talk centered on money, women, work, friends, and the like. Money and cigarette loans were common. There was little use of the swimming pool.

Helen S. was immediately caught up in efforts to make her socialize. More pressure was put on females to interact because they are rare here. Young males immediately started gravitating toward her and engaging her in conversation. I wondered how the other young female residents would react to this newcomer's competition.

As in the mental hospital, success in the board-and-care facility brought me fears of future failure. I compared myself with those who functioned well in spite of their problems. I saw men approach girls, yet I felt incapable of doing so. (In the hospital female nurses and aides were so set apart by their roles that I didn't see them as even potentially accessible companions.) I felt emasculated, frightened, and sometimes lonely. Yet a good blend of friendliness and independence prevailed here. (Among the "15 commandments" posted in the rooms was one asking the patients to welcome newcomers, introduce themselves, and be helpful.) In general, staff attitudes were polite, without showing pity. Concern didn't seem to be phony. I heard "I'm sorry," "Thank you," and other verbal expressions of mutual respect and worth. I resented it when we were called "boys," however, even if the word was used by a motherly staff person.

Showered and went to bed early. Read a little. Slept and had many dreams. In one I taught an oppressed people how to trap and conquer their foes by waiting until the enemy's powerful fleet had committed itself to a narrow channel and then surrounding and blasting it up close while its guns were aimed at distant villages. The analogy to distant therapeutic goals but up close human blindness in our psychiatric institutions seems obvious now. My identification as a leader of patients slipped even into my dreams.

At 12:15 A.M. a fire hydrant across the street was broken and water spurted 25 feet up in the air. A number of residents gathered to watch. "Anyone got a canoe?" I heard. After my initial startled response I looked out the window, saw what was happening, and promptly went back to sleep.

August 8

After breakfast, at 8:15, I went to the facility's bus. I had been told it left at 8:30 but this morning it left at 8:20. One learns to show up for events early and wait — just in case.

It proved to be fairly easy to avoid picking up a routing slip at the VA (usually, residents with jobs pick up these slips so they can get a free lunch and transportation expenses). Then to my assigned "detail" at the Central Research Unit. Back into my David Reynolds identity for a while. Such shifting between identities for extended periods was not a feature of our earlier experiential research. It proved difficult to maintain consistency in either self.

I returned at 2 P.M. for the bus ride back to B Home. The bus was quickly filled. Most of us preferred to wait inside the sun-warmed bus with acquaintances than alone in the fresh air outside. Then we were told we would leave at 3 P.M. that day and 3:15 P.M. thereafter. The reason for the delay was that ex-patients were leaving their jobs too early. "I don't know how long this will last," was the driver's comment. I learned that some patients employed the bus schedule to avoid getting to the hospital in time for group meetings they disliked and as an excuse to leave work early. As we waited, one resident asked me, "Why do they call you 'Doctor'? Is it because of the beard?" I nodded. Perhaps he had heard a social worker who did not know about the project greet me as "Dr. Reynolds."

I lounged in the TV room and so was unable to hear clearly an announcement about the Rustic Canyon Recreation Center. I joined a line impulsively and discovered after a few minutes that it was a pay line. So I went outside and found the bus that was to go to the Recreation Center. After getting on I was worried that perhaps I should have signed up in advance for this outing. I still had no idea whether we were going to a cookout, a therapy group, or whatever. But the timing of the event coincided with my urge to act and there I was. The importance of natural timing is evident here, in having events, activities, greetings, and the like occur when the resident's mood prompts him to take action and to socialize.

The Rustic Canyon setting was a peaceful blend of nature's

artistry and man's. The work with macrame was delayed and disorganized, so there was not enough time to complete the afternoon's project. Residents were not expected to do well, or to care much about what they were doing. Pressures to succeed were minimal. B Home's occupational therapist and the park occupational therapist engaged in private conversations (about business), but they had trouble separating themselves spatially from the residents who followed them around.

The bus returned in time for dinner. On the blackboard in the dining hall was written "Have a nice day!" The houseparents helped to serve the meal, adding a familylike touch. Someone attracted the male houseparent's attention by yelling "Hey." He was reprimanded by a fellow resident: "Not 'Hey'; his name is Jack." The first resident apologized. He hadn't remembered Jack's name.

After dinner I asked for a light bulb and was told to wait in a certain place. "It might take thirty minutes." I waited. After about five minutes I got the bulb because Karl's other job had been completed early. Waiting thirty minutes for a light bulb didn't seem unreasonable in this setting.

I took a walk and bought some doughnuts. The uncensored freedom, a sort of tolerance for unusual behavior, extends to short trips outside the setting as well. I saw fellow residents strolling along the busy boulevard. One I know well was hallucinating as he walked.

The houseparents finished their afterdinner chores and went about greeting residents. The housemother hugged a female resident. Then two guys asked to be hugged. Without hesitation, she did so. "You're all good boys," she reassured them. In this warm motherly context I suppose "boys" is an appropriate term of address and reference. The residents were rather enthusiastic about this demonstration of affectionate concern.

Karl asked me to help carry a crate of empty bottles. The timing was good. I wasn't busy, and I owed him a favor for bringing me the light bulb earlier than promised. This little job wasn't work therapy; it was genuine, meaningful work.

When female residents are present in a setting male behavior takes on a different tone. Chivalry and banter, even among older patients, become an acceptable and enjoyable symbolization of masculinity.

A girl friend (ex-patient) of an agitated female resident came to visit her, keeping an eye on her. It's good to see the role of friend used so positively within this setting. Another resident loaned his friend a dollar with the request that it last him four days.

Some previously meaningful encounters begin to lose their meaning as I get the same introduction and greeting from a patient for the third time or see another one mouth identical phrases to everyone he meets.

There seems to be less talk of food here than in the psychiatric hospital, although such talk isn't absent altogether. There is still a line at the dining room door before meals. But with other things to do and talk about, this topic doesn't have as much import as it did in the hospital.

August 9

Jack is learning to use residents more frequently to perform menial tasks, and the residents recognize and comment on this new work procedure. "Paul, would you do me a favor?" He asks Paul to gather up some empty Coke bottles and put them away. He thanks Paul. Perhaps Paul will learn not to come out of his room before breakfast at 7 A.M. Assigning work to people who sit around is likely to make them spend more time in their rooms or outside the facility.

I rushed in for breakfast near the head of the line, found a seat, and discovered that this morning hot cereal had been placed on a serving cart. Residents grabbed a bowl as they passed. All except me. I didn't know about this custom and had to risk losing my seat to go back for the cereal.

After breakfast, as I sat under the balcony, Jack said, "Good-morning, David." "How are you?" "Fine." These are bittersweet exchanges. Both frightening and pleasing. The timing is important, as are the tone of voice and the naturalness of the encounter.

The newness is wearing off now. Perhaps it wears off faster than usual for me. At any rate, I face the prospect of more of the same, year after year, and the thought is depressing. Two other experiences add to my despondency. One is a comparison of myself with the other persons who live here. One fellow, asked how old he was, responded, "Thirty-seven," and it suddenly struck me that in six years I too might be in the same poor condition he is in. The second factor is that as the status of newcomer wears off people make fewer efforts to express their concern for me (and understandably so, since

I've absorbed so much without returning appropriate responses that would build friendships). And I begin to notice artificiality and stereotyped greetings and selfishness in others. The impact of all these factors gathers force from the expectation that I will be here a long time, perhaps for the rest of my life.

There is little pressure to get the resident out of this board-and-care facility, so what faces him is more of the same. And why should he complain. He has food, shelter, a pool, activities, medication, friends — all within a protected society. The cost, however, includes giving up the respect of the larger society.

Perhaps a predictive therapy would be useful. Much as the Morita psychotherapists in Japan predict the patient's responses to isolated bed rest (Reynolds, 1976), so the aftercare therapist could psychologically vaccinate the resident by warning him of the shock of the encounters he is likely to face in the weeks following his discharge. And in addition to preparing him for discharge, the therapist could encourage him to use his experiences after discharge as benchmarks of progress and as motivation for more community-oriented activities.

On the bus ride back I was struck again by the necessity of catering to Leon's moods. Leon has a way of taking out his depression and anger on residents, though he tries to control this tendency to some extent.

At dinnertime there was no medication envelope for me. Karl intended to get some for me later, but apparently forgot or I wasn't around. The next morning there was again no medication envelope for me.

After dinner I sat outside, reading. Karl asked another resident what was the matter. The fellow said he was in a black depression. Karl told him not to let that bother him. "Do what I do. Shoo your troubles away." Karl takes a self-responsibility approach to disorders. He doesn't put too much stress on this approach, but he does provide a nice balance to the oversympathetic, uncaring, pill-pushing types the residents sometimes meet elsewhere.

The NOVA (New Opportunities for Voluntary Action) meeting began at 6 P.M. in the OT (occupational therapy) room. The issues raised by this ex-mental patient self-help group were well taken. For example, we discussed the NOVA group at another board-and-care establishment which had been forbidden to meet, a retroactive rent increase at some board-and-care homes, and furnishings that were badly in need of repair. Complaints about the meals were overridden by the majority of residents who were satisfied with the food choice and preparation. But as important as the content was the style in which the meeting was run by the B Home of NOVA. The facilitator from outside, Dan, was obviously committed to his task. He wasn't patronizing; he expected residents to behave sensibly. He listened to and rephrased rambling accounts (knowing the members personally helped him to understand what they were trying to say) and politely cut off repetitious meandering. At the same time he deferred to the resident leadership, taking the floor only when necessary, to give background information, relate accounts of recent NOVA activities, offer interpretations of unclear questions, and the like. The setting provided a sense of self-worth and trust and responsibility to the fifteen or twenty residents who attended.

At 7:45 there was an argument at poolside. "Stop bothering me!" one resident kept shouting, and his opponent responded with the same rude remark. The housemother was summoned, and her attempts to placate both parties began with a hug and "You're a good boy" and "It's all right now." Soon she is going to have to learn to set limits, confront residents, and evaluate instigators instead of trying to appease everyone. Her efforts were mildly successful for about thirty seconds, but then the argument broke out afresh. This time two fellow residents, one for each party to the quarrel, came over and calmed them down. Again the mutual cooperation system among residents relieved the pressures of daily life.

At 9 P.M. I made a tour of B Home's night life. There were six or seven people in the TV room and four or five at poolside (where a female resident was kissing her boyfriend). About six men were seated under the balcony, two others were playing table tennis, and one girl was at the phone (she'd been there for at least an hour). In several of the private rooms TV sets were playing.

August 10

Before breakfast, as I sat under the balcony, a man whose ashes had blown onto my trousers brushed them off (actually, he rubbed them in) without saying anything to me. A few residents commented upon one another's appearance; sometimes the remarks were invited, sometimes not.

At breakfast I was struck by the selfishness that is expected behavior at the table. Those who are seated first grab the milk or juice pitcher and pour their own. One resident quickly switched his cereal with that on my plate as he sat down. Again there was no medication for me at the table, but as I left, Don, the administrator, caught me and gave me my pills. He praised my beard.

There was interesting talk about a woman psychiatrist at the VA who the residents suspect is going through change of life. She is too calm. She ought to get excited once in a while. Probably she goes down to the "club" before coming to work. "No telling what *she's* on." "And she tells *us* not to drink!"

"Gee, you're all dressed up this morning." No response at all; the pacing continued. Residents learn that expected responses may not come at all or may be distorted. Thus, when I speak, either I must be somehow self-reinforced for speaking (i.e., I'm a nice guy for saying something, maybe it'll help him to say something, I need to make this comment, etc.) or the saying must be sufficient in itself, not requiring a response. Sometimes remarks are repeated in the hope of eliciting a response.

This morning the bus was late in leaving. We had to wait for Leon. As he pulled out there was an obstacle he wanted to miss. Although we residents told him he was all right, he backed up and pulled out again (not trusting our judgment). He told us to wait up ahead and then stopped the bus back a way so we had to walk over to it. Leon wasn't in a good mood this morning. Several residents called him names under their breath, being careful not to let him hear them.

Three recreation therapists and a couple of residents began cavorting around in the pool. Their unselfconscious play made me think of how different I was, how I wasn't able to participate, how left out I felt. Helen S. came down and watched them for a while, too. I wondered if she felt the same way. I heard an older resident comment on the great difference between himself and these young people.

Then I went to a nearby bookstore, returned, and did some reading by the pool. One resident kept asking Karl to talk with him. Karl claimed he was busy (he'd just finished talking for a few minutes with another resident). The man kept asking each time he saw Karl pass. Karl finally told him to be still, then ordered him to smile: "That's my fine boy." Then he seemed to relent and to be sorry for embarrassing and pressuring the resident, whom he asked to help with a task. And they talked as they worked.

After dinner there was time for wandering around and reading. The schedule posted in the dining room indicated that at 7:30 we were to go to Stoner Park for a weekly dance. I heard no announcement but walked out to the bus. It was almost filled by 7:15. We were expecting to go to a dance, but that night there was a special water carnival instead, and so we attended that. As we waited (and again there wasn't much organization, except that seats were hurriedly saved for groups from several aftercare facilities) some of the residents began to play volleyball. I wandered over to play basketball, and a fellow asked me what all those people were doing over there. I hesitated, but then I realized that he wasn't asking about the group of strange people playing volleyball but about the crowd that had gathered to view the water carnival. I was so sensitive about being a part of what I felt to be a conspicuous and "foreground" group that at first I misinterpreted his question as referring to "us." I was embarrassed to be part of the group, but it was even more upsetting to realize that I depended upon and needed them for my own sense of belonging and of security. To be dependent upon a stigmatized group is disquieting.

The other groups of residents had more young people. One seventeen-year-old girl asked the guys sitting near me to move over so she could sit next to me. She said she was cold and asked if I would keep her warm. She held my hand, asked how old I was, and wanted to know if I had a girl friend and a car. I told her she was too young for me. She took the rejection well and then focused most of her attention on a young man sitting on her other side. Yet she also tried to give me her name, address, and phone number written on a piece of paper. I could handle her only by ignoring, withdrawing from, and diverting her. I suddenly had a panicky feeling that I wasn't ready to handle a relationship, especially with someone who also had problems.

The trip to and from the park was marked by friendly chatter and banter. Almost normal.

Some stray thoughts from the day:

Some residents line up to get food first even if they have no reason to be in a hurry, that is, have nothing in particular to do afterward. It seems to be a competitive urge, a chance to win out over one's fellows. I suspect that those who rush to the head of the food lines would test out differently from their peers on a measure of "need for achievement," despite the severity of their disorders.

Meals are satisfactory here because meat portions are large, eggs are frequently served at breakfast (a fact that has special symbolic import, for some reason, here and in other institutions), real butter and milk are served, and there are unlimited seconds on drinks and bread. Seconds on main dishes can be picked up after everyone else has eaten, I've heard, but it wasn't explained to me, perhaps because I never asked.

This thought brings up the issue of what one knows about the rules and customs of the place. If I don't ask questions, there is much I might never find out. Inquisitiveness and careful watching pay off. So does studied ignorance. For example, Helen tells me that we are expected to make our beds if capable of doing so. No one else ever told me that. I notice that my roommate never makes his bed, so I don't make mine. Every afternoon when I return it has been made for me.

It's surprising how little contact one can have with a person sharing the same room. Beyond daily greetings there's almost no exchange in our room beyond practical questions (such as "What time is it?").

There is plenty of soap and soft toilet paper, and there is no crowding despite the fact that six residents use the same bathroom. Our schedules are different, and not everyone seems to shower here, or even use the toilet. That's a puzzle now.

August 11

Went swimming after return from my "detail." It's hard to act miserable when you're enjoying yourself. The depressed person must use some energy in avoiding situations that will prove enjoyable; that is, he uses energy to protect his depression. No wonder he's tired all the time.

Read science fiction for a while. It adds a new dimension to my experience here. The strangeness of the setting and the released inner controls make other worlds more believable and temporarily "enterable."

After supper went to the Santa Monica Chess Club with Bob (a resident) and lost six straight games to him. He's a former Minnesota state champion. We didn't talk of our mental problems, diagnoses, or medication, although he did mention a physical ailment. He calls B Home a "boardinghouse." In the excursion into society our ex-patient identities were well concealed. Afterward we went to Sambo's for a snack. There are several coffee shop hangouts for the residents and their friends who have cars.

Thoughts on the day:

There is a sort of game involving some patients, staff, and doctors. Among other things drugs help pass the time, so some residents pressure their doctors for more medication. Karl, the person who most closely watches medications, believes that most residents do better on fewer tranquilizers. But, since Karl is in a poor negotiating position, the amount of medication is determined primarily by means of a two-person game between resident and psychiatrist.

There are several types of resident here. One group seems perfectly normal and mature, but with minor physical-neurological impairments. Another group seems highly immature and childish but with no apparent cognitive disruption. They talk about "Daddy," play with yoyos, and cavort around like preteens. Others who are obviously disturbed affectively and cognitively occasionally create social disturbances. Guys and gals who "blow up," shout, and frighten others cause more than fear and temporary upset. They remind us that we are in a place for disturbed people and that we have problems too. Those who pretend the residence is merely a "boardinghouse" must resent the reminder that it is not.

My roommate Edward, was smoking and cracking his knuckles (later I discovered that the noise came from grinding his teeth, not from cracking his knuckles) for at least an hour in the middle of the night. I got up, opened a window, and finally went back to bed and fell asleep. Then, in retaliation, I got up at my usual time of 6:30 and left the light on.

August 12

At breakfast I tried to switch cereals with the resident next to me, but he wanted his own cereal back and I gave it to him. To get even, I passed the milk pitcher to the other end of the table so that he had to ask me politely to pass the milk. Such childishness can be indulged in here.

These petty games indicate that I'm being drawn into social relationships of sufficient depth to cause affective reaction. It is a stage of integration into this society. Before, other people were shadowy factors in my world. Now they are persons to me, and I am no longer a newcomer to this society. To reach this stage may take from a week to a month or more for severely withdrawn patients.

Today I found a small room whose purpose I hadn't realized before. It opens off the TV room and has a table, books, radio, and stereo for resident use. Because I once saw the occupational therapist enter this room, I had assumed it was reserved for staff members. Even after six days here, I'm still picking up simple geographic and logistic information — and I have to look around for it!

This room fills a need I had noted earlier. I thought before that patients had no real personal control over the selection of TV and radio programs (in the bus the driver selects the station and in the TV room one patient tends to dominate, I hear) unless one owned his own radio or TV. This small room however, is used by residents (usually one at a time) to listen to the radio or play their own LP records.

The sign on the wall in my bedroom reads: "Did you forget to take out the trash [we hadn't yet], hang up your clothes [my roommate piles them on a chair], check your appearance [are they kidding?] [and nothing about making the bed].

Karl asked me how the chess club went last night. He had helped arrange it for me. Then he asked if I felt up to helping serve the noon meal. I said I would. This fellow is clever. He generally sets the resident up with a favor and then asks one himself. The other guy who helped serve the noon meal that day had shown up at the office for free soap.

Serving gives a new perspective on meals at B Home. No one asked me to wash my hands. Things were fairly hurried when I came on and perhaps they forgot. For two hours of unpaid menial work we got lots of praise and an early lunch. Hardly worth it in my book. Another guy serving said he does it regularly and gets pocket money for it. The work includes setting the tables, carrying plates of food from the kitchen, cleaning off the tables, and resetting places for the next meal. People were good about explaining simply and not rushing us. Pearl is the chief cook and she obviously runs the kitchen, including the two inexperienced houseparents.

Afterward I went to the music room and played bridge. There's an ingroup of bridge players, and I was adopted immediately, called by my first name, and asked questions about my past and the plans for my future. One player, who is skillful at bridge, asks all sorts of strange questions, one after another: "What is your bridge frequency? — I just wondered"; "Are you the great bridge champion Kent Rosenhoff? — I just wondered." There's idle talk of a tournament. The level of play is fairly high. Everyone is mannerly and sportsmanlike. There's an aura of gentlemanliness, a murmur of quiet conversation, among those who play bridge in the music room.

In bed at 9 P.M., I finally had a confrontation with my roommate as he was lying in bed smoking and staring at the "no smoking in bed" sign on the wall. I told him that smoke gives me a headache, that I'll stay out of the room during the day so he can smoke then. Since I have to come in to sleep I asked him to stop smoking at night. He agreed and soon stopped. Things seem better between us now. It reads like a small thing but it wasn't then.

Thinking back, I see that the resident here, compared with the mental hospital patient, has more options: he picks his friends, he can leave the grounds at will, he can go on scheduled trips, he may own a car, and he may keep all sorts of personal belongings which he couldn't have kept in the hospital. So as my depression lifts there will be more to do when I'm ready to do it — the idea of "natural availability." In fact, I'm beginning to wonder if the "stairstep phenomenon" (success leading to greater fear of bigger failure) which occurred in the hospital may not be associated with success in conjunction with continuing restrictions. Here, success seems to build confidence.

August 13

As I waited for breakfast my recent bridge opponent asked if I was the actor "Somebody-or-other." It's easy to be paranoid about such questions, but I've learned to more or less discount them. It was simply another of Jerry's crazy queries.

I took a nap, shot billiards by myself, and read. All the while I was avoiding Karl, not wishing to get caught again with a work detail. (Once was fine, to see what it was like, for curiosity or science or whatever, but not twice.) It's a fairly effective means of keeping people out of sight during the hour before a meal. Those who sit around in plain sight either don't mind working, haven't learned to stay away, or have a good excuse not to do the work.

Weekends are different from weekdays. There is less to do on the weekends, a smaller staff, and more of a sense of leisure (which is really meaningless because we have so much leisure anyway). That's why the bridge and chess buffs latched on to me. What one does on the weekend depends largely on whether one has a car or no car, relatives or no relatives, friends or no friends, on whether one stays in or goes out, as well as on the level and activity of one's mental state. Phone calls and announcements of visitors over the public address system increase during weekends.

As I sat in the music room before lunch a resident came in and played two melodies on the piano. He played beautifully and professionally for seven or eight minues; then abruptly he got up and left. I wonder if he doesn't do that periodically just to remind himself of who he is. Lunch and then bridge.

Sunday afternoon bingo at 2 P.M. Perhaps twenty patients participated at poolside. Karl led the game and seemed to enjoy joking with the residents and emceeing the game. Prizes were twenty cents to the winner and dimes to the next five or six except for the last game, which netted 40 cents to the winner. Helen S. did well. I won a dime. There were few mistakes. Since Karl couldn't relinquish his other duties while conducting the event, there were several interruptions of four or five minutes while he ran an errand or did a chore. We were expected simply to wait during these delays. During the hour an argument that arose between two residents (a male and a female) led to mutual baiting. The woman called her antagonist "crazy" and a "nut," and through pantomime she made fun of his facial grimace. Clearly she intended to be hurtful. Her tactics revealed the Achilles' heel of the residents, underscoring their usual care to avoid the subject of mental illness in casual conversation. B Home is no retirement facility, no nursing home, no spiritual retreat, no recreation villa; it is a warehouse for society's rejects. We are the cracked eggs, the unfit.

August 14

I'm rather experienced now at portraying various degrees of the "resident shuffle": shoulders slumped, head thrust forward, eyes downcast, slow shuffling gait.

Perhaps one reason that breakfast draws little or no complaint is that residents can order eggs cooked in the style they prefer. We get a feeling of control over this meal.

After breakfast I read, then waited for the bus to leave. Inadvertently I stepped on some oil in the driveway and slipped. I found an old paper bag and began to wipe up the oil. A housekeeper saw me rubbing the torn bag over the cement with my foot. I don't know that she thought I was performing some crazy compulsive ritual but I think she did. Projection or not, when one worries that sensible acts are being taken as insane ones, there's trouble.

Another example of the acceptance of stigma by residents and ex-patients occurred as we waited. One resident was praising another's clothes this morning. "You don't look as if you even belong at the VA," he said. If we are looking to ex-patients to take the lead in reeducating our nation away from prejudice against the formerly mentally ill, we had better look elsewhere. They have learned from professionals a thousand ways to see the disturbed as inferior — and they do.

I find it harder to be depressed around Larry, with whom I play bridge. It may be that because I loosen up a bit at bridge I find it inconsistent to behave in a very depressed manner when I meet Larry, even away from the bridge table. Some might consider him a conditioned stimulus for a nondepressive conditioned response, but I think it's rather an issue of role congruity. Perhaps we need to set up a depressed person in a few positive situations with a pseudotherapist present to share the experience and then to keep the two together for a longer period of time.

When we got back at 3:40 I went to the B Home occupational therapy shop. It was supposed to close at 3 o'clock but Mary, the recreation therapist, was still there playing a game somewhat like Monopoly. She showed me how to finish a macrame project. I appreciate people who help us in either work or play activity beyond official hours. Then a quick swim and letter writing in my room.

I've found a few things to complain about, but, of course, I haven't mentioned them to the authorities. The venetian blinds are filthy, there are roaches in the bathroom, the linen hasn't been changed for a week, and we got margarine for supper tonight.

After supper I played bridge. There wasn't much that I liked at supper, so I went on a doughnut binge at a nearby shop. It would be revealing to ask residents to draw maps of the area around B Home. Taco places, ice cream parlors, bars, the doughnut shop, and bus stops would probably be well documented, comparatively speaking.

At about 7:00 I returned and heard the last few minutes of an argument between a young female resident and a visitor. Don, the manager, was handling this situation with confident control.

I forgot my key and asked Jim, the housefather, to let me into my room. I felt bad and apologized. He said he didn't mind "this time" but told me not to forget my key late at night, when I'd have to wake him up and he'd have to let me in the outer doors, too. Failure still builds feelings of worthlessness in me out of all proportion to the stimulus.

The other day I felt free enough to get up and say to the guy who was to be a fourth at bridge that I didn't like to play with beginners (he'd just told us he'd never played the game), and I walked away. Now he and his girl friend (she's not really his girl friend, from her point of view) avoid me and show no friendliness because they think I'm a snob. In other words, the freedom to behave spontaneously in this place has social consequences. When I use the freedom I must sometimes pay later in esteem and other social rewards.

August 15

I recall that last night after Helen left the canteen someone asked who she was. "Helen, Helen of Troy," was another resident's reply. And, oh, yes, after the maid cleaned my room there was one of my hidden yellow Elavil pills on the floor. No repercussions.

My weekdays are divided into scheduled waiting periods: from getting up until breakfast, after breakfast until the bus leaves, duty assignment, from getting back until supper, after supper until bedtime. These routine time periods are starting to be filled by predictable activity. For example, after supper usually comes bridge, before breakfast comes washing up, dressing, and reading or note writing. It will be interesting to see how regularized, that is, how structured, these activities become after two or three weeks.

This morning fifteen people sat around the TV room. News was on, but no more than five people were watching or listening. Others dozed or stared ahead. The chairs are comfortable there.

On the bus one resident remarked that B Home is better than the hospital because there are too many crazy people in the hospital and you have to put up with too much crazy talk.

At work, especially, but also at B Home I'm beginning to notice a change in my behavior. I'm becoming more impulsive, more concerned with immediate gratification. It's hard to concentrate on writing. I have urges to eat (particularly doughnuts and ice cream) and I indulge them rather freely. I think more about activities per se and less about their long-term purposes or consequences. Perhaps these changes are a reaction to the long periods of waiting at the board-and-care home. Perhaps they are a response to the lessening of responsibilities and the weakening of purpose in this particular life style.

Returning on the bus we stopped for gas. One patient was smiling and waving at the station attendant, a stranger, who was smiling and nodding back. When asked what he was doing, the resident said, "He thinks *I'm* crazy, and I think *he's* crazy."

I recognize a mood cycle that occurs spontaneously. I can "ride it" into a deeper depression or out of the depression as it occurs. It provides impetus but not always in the desired direction.

Albert, my roommate, told me he would give me the dollar I loaned him yesterday on the first of September instead of today, as he'd promised. I said I might not be around then. He replied that if I was gone he would send it by mail.

I wanted to go to crafts at Rustic Canyon but the group had already left. This incident is another example of not knowing what is routine and what is not. Last week we were back from the VA in time to go.

Today our sheets are clean (at least one sheet is — Larry says they put the top sheet on the bottom and put a clean one on top), but the towels are unchanged.

August 16

When he got to the VA to pick us up Leon asked for three volunteers to help carry packages up to a ward. I helped, worrying that someone might recognize me. The nurse in charge thanked Leon at the completion of the task but ignored us. On the bus ride back Karen, a young resident, teased Leon that she had something on him that would get him into trouble if she told, but she didn't mention what it was. He asked her if she'd like to see her nineteenth birthday!

There were clean towels when we arrived back at B Home. We got one towel each but no washcloths (though they are provided in other rooms).

As I was swimming I heard two residents refuse to work in the kitchen that evening. One had an appointment elsewhere and the other just didn't feel like it. They weren't pressured further. It is said that we do not need to help out with the chores if we don't want to, but one wonders if little favors might be harder to elicit from the staff if we refuse to cooperate.

6:00 P.M. NOVA meeting. I like Dan, the NOVA organizer who seems to feel we are capable of dealing collectively with some of our life problems. There is the sense that Don, Mary, and Leon don't have a very high opinion of residents' capacities. Although they are competent, professional, and even interested staff members, they don't see the common human and social needs of the residents. Leon in particular is at times jovial, helpful, and in confident control of things, but he is so self-centered and so walled off from the residents that he almost radiates differentness from us. I would speculate that he's either an ex-patient who needs to emphasize his difference or a former nursing assistant with the same needs.

At the NOVA meeting the topic of eviction came up. Although owners can apparently evict residents without notice, residents must give owners fifteen days' notice if they want to leave. The legality of this arrangement is currently in question. There were complaints about the meat patties served that evening and praise of the field trip that day. It is noteworthy that events like the field trip generate a lot of normal conversation. Those who went have something to talk about.

August 17

Albert woke up coughing this morning. I saw him after breakfast and asked how he was. He said he'd probably have to get X rays. I suggested he might get some medicine for his cough. He paid me the dollar he owed me.

Found roaches in my chest of drawers and in the bathroom. Told Jack who sent me to Don. Don said he'd have the exterminators come to our apartment this morning.

I've been thinking that if NOVA wants to apply pressure to boarding homes it isn't necessary to go to state licensing authorities, but simply to organize sympathetic social workers. If there are no referrals, there is no profit for board-and-care facilities.

We were told several days in advance that we would leave early today for the VA so the bus could be serviced at 8:30. We are made to feel that B Home is doing us a favor by providing transportation. The bus was crowded, and Leon told some passengers to take public transportation today and others to start doing so tomorrow. Leon said that if B Home bought a larger bus it would soon be filled, too. It is his tone rather than what he says which makes Leon's speech so offensive. There is a sadistic "God-how-you-guys-are-a-burden" quality to his interactions with male residents. The women get somewhat gentler treatment.

When we returned, Don and the secretary were splashing around in the pool. There was lots of touching, and there were innuendos, but no obvious improprieties. They were in the pool for forty-five minutes after we returned. Don remarked in response to a resident's comment that just because he's the manager doesn't mean he doesn't like to swim. Sandy, a young female resident, was teasing him. He grabbed her and threatened to throw her into the pool. She screamed but bluffed and dared him to go ahead, knowing he wouldn't. And he didn't.

After supper I played bridge. Everyone knew Jerry wouldn't play that night. He begins preparing early for the dance. He was ready by 6 P.M. and had to wait an hour for the bus.

At the dance the recreation leaders enjoyed themselves. The residents did the best they could. We all had a good time. For a while we forgot who we were. The ride back was festive and cheerful — or was I projecting?

August 18

At pickup time at the VA, an old fellow who was coming to B Home for the weekend waited with us. If he liked the place he'd come back on Thursday to stay. He asked a lot of questions, as a newcomer has to do, and was told by the other residents that he'd probably like B Home. He was taken on the usual tour upon arriving and before supper had time for a beer down the street.

After supper the newcomer pumped me for more information, and I even volunteered some, especially about medication procedures. I'm new too, and new people like to display their knowledge. I find myself drawn to people who seem worse off than I am. The comparison gives me a feeling of competence.

When I came back to our apartment to shower and change a woman was talking to a resident in the first room. I often walked around my underwear since it never dawned on me that women could come into our apartment. Later I discovered that men go into women's apartments too. It's permitted, I guess.

I was restless, waiting to see if Bob's car was fixed. Then he would decide whether he felt like going to the chess club. I don't like depending so heavily on uncontrollable events to determine my activities. I wandered from canteen to TV room to poolside to my room and around the circuit again. There's a suggestion box on the TV set with a stack of questionnaires about preferred foods underneath. I filled one out yesterday, marked it, and put it into the box. We'll see how long it remains. It's still there — all by itself.

Don talked with Karen and Brooks for a while and then Karen went sobbing into her room with the other two trailing behind. They talked (the blinds carefully opened) until nearly 9 P.M. Don and Leon are trying to do some sort of psychotherapy with the girls who live here. I wonder how proficient they are. I note a personal sense of frustration that I am not allowed to help. I could only pace around and worry about what was bothering Karen. She wants help from Don, not from me, and their talking is carried out more or less privately. After all, when the choice comes, one's fellow residents aren't as qualified to help as "normals."

To bed and asleep by 9. After I'd been asleep for perhaps an hour, Albert came in, switched on the lights, and asked if he could borrow a dollar until Tuesday because he had eaten too much and needed to get something to drink. I handed him a dollar without a word. Good grief!

August 19

Albert was up early drinking soft drinks. Leon caught him and scolded him for breaking his ulcer regimen. Leon told Albert he'd have to sign himself back into the hospital on Monday because this sort of thing had gone on for too long. Later Albert was outside coughing and Leon ordered him back into his room.

The fellow who's usually at the head of the meal line was there again this morning. Last night someone else got there about an hour early just to be ahead of him. There was teasing, which led to harsh words, and the two men almost got into a fight. The one who likes to be first in line is a stooped, ineffectual old fellow, and this game is one of the few he wins.

Brian comes in smiling. He describes how he was yelled at, hit, and kicked by his ex-roommate Ken. This is the fourth time it has happened. Brian moved to a different room, Jerry's, two weeks ago. The smile is to let us know he's all right, but it also signifies an event, something that sets Brian off. This Saturday is now special.

Leon and Jack go over to talk to Ken. I tell Jerry about his current roommate's injuries. Leon returns. Jerry says, "I hear my roommate was hit." Leon evades the issue, asking "Is that so?" Then Leon spots Brian. "You can go back now. He won't hurt you. Go over and he'll apologize. Next time I wish you'd hit him back." "If you hit him back you wouldn't end up causing me so much trouble" is Leon's implied message. A black resident goes up to Brian and says, "Look, when a man hits you you're supposed to hit him back."

The resident in the next room still spends the day in bed — except for meals.

I decided to talk to Don. I went up to the office but Don wasn't there. So I sat in a chair waiting for Leon to finish filling out some papers with another resident. I told Leon of my guilt feelings about taking up space on the crowded bus. "I don't want you to feel guilty about that," he said, explaining that some of us aren't capable of taking public transportation. When I am ready to do so, he told me, it will be a step forward. I also told him that I felt guilty about lending Albert a dollar when I discovered he bought Cokes with it. Leon slipped easily into a fatherly adviser role. What I do with my money is my own business ("It's up to you"), but some people don't have the willpower to stay away from things that hurt them. And you don't always get your money back. He said he'd lent money that had never been returned.

Then I told him I'd probably leave at the end of the month. I had already talked to my social worker about it. "That's fine. It's a step forward for you." The words were acceptable, but it seemed to me that he was parroting what he was supposed to say. Then he thanked me. "I appreciate your coming in."

Leon turned and barked angrily at a man for tapping on the office window. "Don't ever do that again!" Then he switched immediately and gave a friendly smiling response to another man's greeting.

Bridge until 1:30. Jerry continues to talk irrationally at times, but he keeps equating me with actors and today asked me if I was Doctor Somebody. He followed that query by asking if I was married to Helen Summers. He seems to be sensitive to cues of which we aren't aware. Fortunately for our research, no one takes his ramblings seriously.

My roommate asked for a dime but I refused, telling him I knew he'd spend it on a soft drink that isn't good for him.

Helen went out again today. It must be hard for her never having been in the service and so never having acquired the knack of marking time and immersing herself in routine. I take pleasure in showering, selecting clothes, dressing, and even in waiting for the next event (like supper).

5 P.M. Supper. Each person who opens the divider that allows us to enter the dining hall does so in a characteristic way that communicates his feelings about us. For example, Flo says, smiling, "Come on in, boys." It's as if she's happy to feed us. Jack silently, rather grimly, opens the door wide, as if it's only a job he has to do. Others joke about the rushing horde, the stampede, or the rush hour. By making fun of our eagerness to eat, they put themselves above us.

August 20

Up at 6:30. Shaved. Albert got up a few minutes before I left. Who would speak first this morning? Neither of us.

Talked to Jerry before breakfast. He asks if I know my jumping-off point, my no-turning-back point, my stair number, and on and on. I can relate many of my recent thoughts to these questions. The possibility of extrasensory perception is rather intriguing. How suggestible I've become!

Then I walked to a nearby church. I'd never gone to this kind of church before, and so familiarity with the service wouldn't affect my impression of it. The songs and some of the worship service were recognizable. But what stood out were the warm greetings at the close of the service. I was seen as another human being, another worshiper. No one knew I was an ex-patient or that I was living at B Home. I felt accepted in a different social world.

Then, at 1:20, came bingo. The caller of the bingo game, a resident named White, was arousing a lot of antagonism by his slow methods. Someone called Leon, who brusquely told White not to check the cards but to give dimes to all who said they won. Shortly afterward, as he sat in the sun, White suffered a severe epileptic seizure. No one touched him as he lay on the ground. Everyone yelled for Leon. No panic. Leon came and checked the man's tongue, finally sending someone for an ambulance when a second seizure started. Leon kept things under calm control. The only errors were minor ones: he failed to protect White's bare skin from being burned on the hot concrete and he did not shield White's eyes from the sun. (I did both.) Calm suggestions from others to call the ambulance and to raise White's head were acted on smoothly. Actually, the fire department rescue squad came. Then they called for the ambulance, which arrived quickly.

After a few minutes hot chocolate and rolls were served by the pool with Leon helping. He had all of us who played bingo line up and get dimes in lieu of finishing the game. An inexpensive payoff.

Thinking over the two weeks I've been here, I realize that some comments need to be added to this journal. Some have to do with what did *not* happen. No one on the staff approached me to get me to talk, but staffers were willing to listen to me if I took the initiative. No effort was made to match me with an appropriate roommate; the policy seems to be to fill in where there's a vacancy and then, if a serious problem arises, to switch roommates. There is nothing much here for a bright, lively person. Perhaps there are few such people in these settings, but the atmosphere stifles rather than stimulates the mind.

August 21

I overheard a resident asking to borrow Don's key. Don replied, "No. sir; that's what you get for forgetting yours."

Why do my friendships here seem less intimate than those in the psychiatric hospital? Perhaps we ex-patients are less desperate for human contact, less accepting of one another's idiosyncrasies. Perhaps we have more time here and more options for choosing companions from among our fellow residents. Perhaps the friendship possibilities outside the home lessen the intensity of the need for friends inside it. Perhaps we don't experience the suffering and constriction that foster camaraderie as a defense.

Mario didn't get up for the bus ride to the VA. When Don asked if everyone was present, somebody said that Mario was missing. Don got out and went back inside. The fellow who informed Don about Mario's absence was told that he should not have said anything. "M.Y.O.B." "Never volunteer for anything." "If Mario had wanted to go he would have been here." These comments were being made while Don was gone. No one will make the same "mistake" again. When Don returned he said nothing about the delay, nothing about Mario. Worthwhile people deserve explanations; we didn't.

I felt a bit low this morning, partly because I didn't get medication last night (even though I never take it) and so I expected to feel bad. Medicine, for some of us, is something we *deserve*. We may even jockey for more of it. "They" must bring it to us. It is a symbol of our worth.

When Karl drove up in the bus at 3:25 we felt free to ask him why he was late, and he replied from a defensive position. We couldn't take this stance with Leon or Don. There was lighthearted, even silly, joking on the bus ride back.

When we returned I went to the recreational therapy room. A resident named Wendel came over and talked with me about his plans for leaving B Home and about his former suicidal behavior. He spoke knowledgeably about Prolixin, Ritalin, Thorazine, Mellaril, and "psychic energizers." He had done some pretty bad things in his life, he felt, and he said his only chance for getting into heaven was to claim insanity! Thus he can't afford to get well, for to recover would have eternal consequences for him.

After dinner I played Ping-Pong with Helen. Sam, a resident, came up and whispered that Helen wants to be "had" by me and advised me on how I should go about it. Then, as I watched Helen play a game with Pinkus, Sarge wanted to know if Helen is a virgin. He thought so from watching her dance last Thursday. I told him to ask her — I didn't know. Finally he asked her how old she was and if she was a virgin or not. She was embarrassed and blew a few points in the Ping-Pong game.

I played and won a couple of games of pool from Mike; then I talked with Helen for about half an hour. She had broken a toe last night while I was away from B Home. The time she needed me I wasn't around. I felt bad about it, even though it was an unpredictable event.

I told Karl I'd be leaving B Home. He took the news casually, almost distinterestedly, saying he would make a note that I would be leaving about September 1. I plan to stay until the third.

Then I helped Jerry do his laundry. He can't count change, tell time, or read. We have begun to show him how to do these things for himself.

Then a shower and to bed. My roommate is back from the VA. He was right; they didn't keep him there. They changed his medication but, as usual, he walked around drinking Cokes all evening. Self-destruction, perhaps, but also rebellion and attention seeking; furthermore, he likes soft drinks.

Afterward I told Jack that there are still cockroaches in our bedroom and bathroom. He said Don was around somewhere, but he didn't know if I'd be able to find him. I asked if Don was in Karen's apartment. He said, "Yes," but added that if I knocked Don probably wouldn't answer. Shortly afterward Don came out and I told him about the roaches. He was surprised that the exterminators hadn't taken care of the problem. He had left a note for them, he said. "Thanks for telling me, Kent. If there's anything bothering you, anything at all, you let me know about it." The implication seemed to be that roaches are in the category of things that "bother" me: roaches, suicidal thoughts, delusions, and the like. I felt as if there was something odd about my being bothered by roaches.

As I lay in bed I thought of a parable that aptly describes this board-and-care home. And I dreamed I was schizophrenic.

> Once upon a time there was a flock of 150 sheep, divided into two flocks with several shepherds watching over them. Sometimes a sheep would change suddenly into a dragon and all the other sheep would cower and run to the shepherds because the dragon-sheep hurt other sheep. The shepherds were strong and skillful at rounding up dragon-sheep and sending them to a protected place until they changed back into sheep again. And peace reigned again in the flock.
>
> There were a few lambs in the flock. They were beautiful to behold and the shepherds spent a disproportionate amount of time with them. A few sheep grumbled about being neglected, but not too loudly because they didn't want to be mistaken for dragon-sheep and put away. And many sheep simply didn't care who got the shepherds' attention, provided they had grass and long days to nibble at it and a place to rest at night.
>
> But the pastures for the sheep grew old and dry with time. Insects and dirt blew over them and damaged the land. And some sheep raised a cry: "Help us, shepherds; make our pastures green and beautiful again. We deserve your care." A few bold ones bleated, "We demand your care!" But shepherds have many interests. They have their own families; they must make a profit in their business; they have their own lives to live; they have their special lamb-pets.

I wonder . . . Do sheep ever stampede?

In my dream I hallucinated an interesting, unusual, but orderly world. In the mental hospital, with treatment, the real world gradually superimposed itself on my imagined world and finally took over. But the real world, so mundane and full of complex characters, was complicated and sordid and aesthetically unpleasing. The loss of the imagined world was tragic, and I felt quite alone and lost for a while after coming awake. Soon I was dreaming again.

In this dream I became the leader of a movement to hire schizophrenics for particular jobs that use their skills. For example, they were able to spot a new radar blip on a screen full of blips and to see interference more quickly than a "normal." They worked shorter shifts but with more efficiency because they weren't bored by the repetitious blip patterns on the screen.

August 22

I discovered a barber shop next door to my room. It has a barber's chair and equipment. The door was opened and I looked in. Who uses it? When?

At dinner there was a tranquilizer capsule on the floor of the dining room.

I find myself more and more drawn to the "well" people and the staff. It becomes less natural for me just to sit among those who are less communicative. The sense of time here is rather like that in the service or in the hospital. There's a lot of time, and it's less of a concern in structuring one's day, except that it needs to be filled somehow. I heard a chap on the bus say that he stayed off his detail one day a week to catch up on his rest and to get his clothes in order. But the detail (including the bus ride) lasts only from 8:15 to 3:30 and he has weekends free. Time in such abundance sometimes results in one's doing less, because there's plenty of time to do things later. Our bridge and chess games are rarer now. At first we jumped at this way of filling time, but we overdid it. I became tired of the games. And the music room is stifling on a hot evening.

My roommate isn't cracking his knuckles constantly, I've discovered. He's grinding his teeth.

I went in to watch television before bed, hoping that I wouldn't run into too many people who would ask questions about my leaving. I've been trying to talk individually with everyone I know fairly well. Somehow, it's even harder with people I never really knew. If this business of leaving is so hard after one month, what must it be like after a couple of years?

August 23

An agitated, depressed resident told me he wakes up relaxed, but after he paces for a while he begins to get tense. And time goes slowly for him when he paces. He used to be able to read to pass time; now he can't sit still long enough to read. He goes to movies, making the rounds of different theaters on a regular, planned circuit.

I found a roach in the bathroom. It's hard to describe the feeling of impotence and anger. All I can do is ask for help and all I get is reassurances. I slept with angry fantasies on my mind.

At 3 A.M. my roommate lit a cigarette. "You shouldn't do that," I told him sleepily. He took his time finishing the cigarette. A few minutes later he lit another. I felt he was trying to "get to me." "That does it!" I jumped up and hastily threw on my clothes, shouting at him: "I'll raise hell and see if you keep this up." I stalked over to Jack's apartment, rang the bell, and got him out of bed. I complained about my roommate's noise and the smoking. Jack said, "I can't do anything about his grinding his teeth, but you tell him that in the morning I'll report the smoking to Don." I gave the message to my roommate, and he stopped smoking immediately. Then it dawned on me I was lying only a few feet away from an angry, frustrated former mental patient. Was it safe to go back to sleep while Albert stalked out of the room, came back in, banged his headboard against the wall, and glared at me? I lay with one eye half open, watching, but trying not to look as if I expected him to do anything violent. If something dangerous was going to happen it should happen soon. After half an hour I fell asleep. Later I learned that Albert had gone after his previous roommate with a straight razor. Glad I didn't know about his attack at the time.

August 24

I told Don at breakfast that I needed to talk with him. A few minutes later I was waiting as he came into the office. I was angry. "What's on your mind, Kent?" "I haven't given you any trouble, have I?" "No, you haven't. In fact, you're an asset to the place." "The roaches you said you'd take care of are still there." "The exterminator was in yesterday," he told me and showed me the bill. "Well, I killed one last night." "I'll call them up again," he promised. In the same angry tone, pacing, I complained about the roommate who grinds his teeth and smokes all night. He offered to move me that evening to another room. I said fine; any change would be welcome.

"How long are you going to be here, Kent?" Don asked me then. "Until the third." "I like you, Kent [hand on my shoulder]. I've seen you walking around the pool talking to people. We'll miss you. If you ever need to come back I want you to know you're welcome here. If you need anything call Keith [my social worker] or me anytime. I don't mean that you are to think of returning as a crutch. Go out and give it the old college try on the outside. But if you decide to come back just let us know."

That afternoon Albert inquired, "You moving?" "Yeah." "Hasta la vista," he replied, unconcerned. After the move, Karl thought I might not leave after all.

I tend to be more quiet and more careful around authority figures than I am with fellow residents, because I realize that the former wield more power over my life. My caution may be mistaken for withdrawal. An adequate estimation of a person's mental state may be possible only when he's observed interacting with familiar peers.

A new resident, Chris, rang the apartment bell. He had forgotten his key. He seemed to be a rather far-out, quiet, soft-spoken youth. He started to leave again without taking his key, but I reminded him and he took it. A few minutes later he was back ringing the bell. I opened the door. He was standing there, key in hand. We talked about his being new here and I said he would get used to the place after a while.

I went to bed for the third time. Chris came over to the side of my bed in his shorts and stood there for a moment before going to bed. A few minutes later there he was again, standing beside my bed. In a flat voice he asked, "Want a blow job?" "No, thanks," I replied, trying to act as if he'd offered me a stick of gum. "Go back to bed, man." Soon he was up wandering around. "Look, we can't have you wandering around all night. Some of us have to go to work in the morning." He muttered that he wasn't "set right." I said we'd try to help him get well. Then he lit a cigarette in bed and I showed him the posted rules about that. "I don't want to sound as if I'm laying a lot of rules on you, but you'd better adapt to them once and for all, and then you'll fit in fine."

Paul, another roommate, rang the bell a little later. Groaning, I rose and opened the door. "Don't tell me you were still up," Paul remarked. "No, I wasn't; I had to get up to answer the door." He said I shouldn't talk smart. I muttered that he'd asked me if I was asleep and I had told him I wasn't. "You won't tell Brian on me, will you?" he asked. "No, I won't," I said, but I had no idea what he was talking about. In about half an hour I finally got back to sleep after Paul and Chris had stopped mumbling, shouting, and tossing about. So ended a couple of difficult nights.

August 25

I got up at 6. The sheets on the bed in my room hadn't been clean the night before so I had doubled the top sheet over and slept between the folds. This morning I changed the dirty linen with that from my former bed. Tried to wake Chris for breakfast at 6:45 but he merely mumbled with eyes wide open and then went back to sleep.

I ate only a little breakfast and skipped out before medications. It's 7:20 and I'm writing this "letter." I told Don about last night's proposition from Chris. Said it didn't bother me because he wasn't insistent, but I felt it might trouble Paul if Chris spoke to him the same way.

This morning as we waited for the bus to leave, Mack B, the owner of B Home, drove up. "Hi, Mack," several guys greeted him in a casual friendly manner. He seems to be well liked and not such an authoritarian figure after all.

On the bus ride to the VA this morning Ed remarked how much he liked B Home. No one responded one way or the other, but the silence was rather informative.

Still no mention of my failing to take the medication handed to me at meals. I've accumulated enough Elavil to do damage should I decide to do so. It's hidden in my shaving kit. If we are supposed to be responsible for taking medicine, why do they dole it out?

Ed noted that John doesn't shave or bathe often enough. John became quite upset on hearing the criticism, and Ed recognized the problem instantly. I'm not making fun of you, John," he explained. "I'm just giving you some advice." He knew it was necessary to protect John's ego.

Ernie was sitting by the weights as I worked out between dips in the pool. He suggested a couple of exercises. Then we talked about his former job of lifting kegs and cases of beer for a trucking company. His thoughts and speech sometimes drift and his voice becomes unnaturally soft, but what he says is usually intelligible. When I went back in swimming he offered to keep an eye on my wallet and watch for me. Since our talk he's greeted me warmly whenever we meet. Ernie has been at B Home nearly three years and obviously intends to stay.

At dinner I grabbed the punch and poured a glass for myself even before I sat down. I beat even those two cooperating residents this time. As Karl passed the table he remarked, "Oh, Kent, we moved that little fellow from your room." "Oh." (So long, Chris.)

Bob came by unexpectedly and asked if I wanted to go to the chess club tonight. It's a special treat to learn that something extraordinary will be injected into an otherwise ordinary evening. We entered the world of normals at the club and at a restaurant afterward, returning after midnight.

I found my paperback science fiction book lying on a table in the patio as I passed through. It reminded me of all the things I'd been forgetting lately — my sweater (perhaps it's on the bus or at my detail), my keys (misplaced twice), books, swim trunks in the bathroom, and so forth. My mind continues to function in a distracted manner here. David Kent is particularly bothered by these lapses; he interprets them as indications that he is on the way to becoming a Jerry or a George or a John. Staying at B Home is safe and easy but it's a step on that path, too. So I feel forced to leave this facility before I'm ready because later on I'll be even less ready.

As I withdraw a bit this morning, lying in bed, the sounds of activity outside my room mock me and emphasize the difference between me and others. How can they care so little, to be able to go on with their lives while I am sad, not even wondering why I'm not among them? Such is the self-centeredness of the depressed.

Paul (with five or six others) was sitting in the stair lobby as I passed through last night heading for bed. He tried to engage me in some insane abstract philosophical ramblings. I begged out on grounds of sleepiness, but he followed me up to our room. I insisted

I'd understand it better in the morning. He got hurt and angry and said he could hardly wait until Tuesday so he could talk with his social worker (as if to say social workers listen and understand, even though you won't). Then he was in and out, turning lights on and off the next couple of hours. I checked my watch at 2:30, and saw that he was finally getting into bed.

August 26

Up at 7. Shaved. Went to breakfast. Don called me "David" instead of "Kent" as he passed out medication. Perhaps he likes me. There's a soft quality to his voice when he speaks to David Kent. Soothing.

From 7:30 until 9 writing these "letters" in my room. It is necessary to note that my bowel movements again parallel my depression course as they did when I lived in a psychiatric hospital as a depressed researcher-patient. On first arriving here I became constipated, but the problem gradually became less severe as my spirits improved. Constipation may be a function of the dimension of inactivity-activity in part, but not altogether because I was more active from the start here than I was during the entire mental hospital study, yet the degree of constipation, has been about the same. I do not recall being constipated as an adult except for these two times. I must be the anal-retentive depressed personality type. As support for his theory, Freud would love it!

The middle-class auto-addicted Californian might be surprised at the area one can cover in only an hour's walk. Some B Home residents do a great deal of walking. I recall waving to one of them who was waiting at a bus stop a couple of miles from B Home as we drove to the chess club last night. It's comforting to see familiar faces when I venture out from this place. They, too, are wayfarers.

Jerry came by and asked, "Is Helen Summers your future wife? Do you wish to get married?" I laughed and told him to ask her. He insists I'd make a good part-time instructor — in bridge, chess, weight lifting — at B Home; he'd say anything to keep me around to play chess and bridge with him after I move.

Jerry's "off-the-wall" question for everyone today was, "If God granted you three wishes, what would they be?" Most people said they would have to think about it, but John — mumbling, hallucinating, and word-salad-speaking John — came out with a most insightful wish for himself: "Being understood."

Karen is worried that Don will leave her just as her mother once left her. She learned that he is going away on a vacation. They'll talk about it later.

Jimmy was exiled from home because he chased his father out of the house with a butcher knife and got into other kinds of trouble. He went to County General Hospital, was sent to Camarillo State Hospital, and ended up here. He has been waiting all day for his mother to pick him up and take him home for a visit. He plans to surprise her with his new clothes. (She never came.)

A chartered bus came at about 6:45 to pick us up for the big Western roundup dance. Almost all of us climbed aboard even though we knew it was too early. We didn't want to take a chance on being left behind. There was much confusion about what other stops the bus would make on the way to Friendship Hall in Hollywood. Jerry said he had heard that we were supposed to pick up residents at another board-and-care home on the way. Don was skeptical, but Jerry kept insisting until finally we drove there, Don still kidding Jerry and unbelieving. Jerry was right. Later, when Don and Mary asked how many residents from the other facility had boarded the bus, one B Home resident told them there were four. Nevertheless, Don and Mary counted for themselves without later acknowledging that the resident had been right. His counting hadn't counted.

All in all, however, staff and resident do respond to rational behavior. When I behaved sensibly people put some confidence in me despite my labeled status. And on the few occasions when I thought they were not responding satisfactorily to sensible behavior, I felt compelled to behave irrationally and with anger in order to gain my end, to restore balance, to get even, to correct the unjust "tilt." In this sense, too, others can "drive you crazy."

During the bus ride Don and Mary talked just with each other. Don was engaged in hustling Mary, but only halfheartedly and in a half-joking manner. They talked of Chris's not being well enough to be out of the hospital. Not only were we nonpersons excluded from their conversation, but we were ignored, and thus we overheard things best spoken of privately.

At the roundup there was much evidence of lack of planning. Someone collected fifty cents at the door. Then they returned the money to some of us who arrived later but not to those already there. And the band was late. The Western theme was apparent in the dress of a few people (almost exclusively staff members) and in the paper name tags cut in the shape of sheriff's stars.

The dance was disappointing. Perhaps eighty people attended.

Most of them were old people who simply sat the whole evening at long tables along the sides of the room. The refreshments were an orange drink and cookies (no sandwiches, as promised). The men from B Home joked about the scarcity of unescorted girls. Bobby, for example, directed complaint after complaint to me. Yet at the end of the evening, as Bobby got off the bus, Don asked him if he had a good time, and he responded with oily effusiveness that he'd had a fine time.

The young performers in the band laughed at some of the dancers. At intermission they shouted out to one another to be careful: "It's catching." They played well, however. Their musicianship eclipsed their humanity.

During the dance I sat alone for the most part, focusing on how different and how isolated I am from the others. But I ate more than half a dozen cookies and enjoyed listening to the music and watching the dancing. Although the evening was a mixture of enjoyment and disappointment, I can emphasize either — and David Kent concentrates on the latter.

I asked Mary whether she thought I was ready to leave B Home. Doubts about leaving have begun to arise. She said she didn't know me very well, though she thinks I'm a likable guy. She said it's up to me to decide when to leave; she doesn't know what's in my head, nor does she know why I went to the hospital and why I came to B Home. I told her the suicide attempt story. She warned that I will face difficult problems on the outside, though there will also be good times. It's the same for everyone. The outcome depends on how you react to difficulties. It will be pretty lonely sometimes, she thought. Her tone was concerned, and it lacked artificial "therapizing."

In this journal I haven't meant to be overly critical of the staff at B Home. At times Don and Leon and (especially) Mary treated us as fellow humans and showed genuine concern and a desire to help. Don is likeable in spite of his affected heartiness, but both he and Leon (and Mary, too, to a lesser degree and in a different way) have walled themselves off from involvement (with male residents at least) by a kind of pseudoprofessionalism that comes from having "been around." It is rumored that Don was promoted to manager from the recreation therapist position. I'm reminded of the folk understanding in the armed forces that officers who come up from the enlisted ranks are often more uptight and severe than those who start out as officers. The former always feel a little uncomfortable about their progression upward and need to remind themselves and others of their importance.

August 27

I find today that what I miss most has been activities emphasizing privacy and independence. In other times and other identities I especially enjoyed cooking for myself, watching television programs that I myself wanted to see, listening to my own choice of records, and enjoying the quiet and the freedom of movement in my apartment, alone.

Today Jimmy was excited about a purse snatching. One of our female residents was on her way to the doughnut shop when her purse was grabbed. She stood screaming while the thief ran off down an alley. The purse contained ten dollars and her key. She was especially worried about losing her key, but Don gave her another one. Later she asked Jimmy and another male resident to escort her back to the doughnut shop because she was afraid to go alone.

August 28

Up at 6:15. At 6:50 the door to the TV room was opened and twenty of us pushed our way inside.

Leon is grouchy this morning. "John, don't do that in here." John was playing his endless ball game in the TV room. "Wait a minute!" Leon barks at another man who asks him a favor. "Would you please count to 50 and hold your breath." The tone lets us know that Leon isn't to be pushed today.

At poolside Bobby calls out, "Good-morning, Tom." "Good-morning." "You know my name — [it's] Bobby." Whether one greets another by name or not is important here, too.

As we rode to the VA in the bus there was talk about a couple of guys who slept all day under the covers with their shoes on. Sleeping seems reasonable enough at B Home — "There's nothing to do all day" — but not under the blanket with one's shoes on.

Ed, the former alcoholic, told us that he planned to visit a prostitute on payday. The last time he went it cost him $20 and at the moment he doesn't have that kind of money. The same theme was picked up again on the way back. Someone offered to fix up a couple of guys with a gal who "goes down" for money. She's a divorced waitress, thirty-five years old, who lives in West Los Angeles with her two children. She needs the money. Ed said he had $5 but would prefer to do it on credit. Her "sponsor" responded, "I can't ask that; she's a friend of mine." There was talk of difficulty "getting it up" while taking the tranquilizer Mellaril, of a $50 shot, a $150 "all-nighter" in Las Vegas, and a $1,000 week with a "broad" in Leon's youth. Stu whispered righteously to me, "Now we're getting to see how the other half lives."

Went swimming and did weight lifting until dinner. After dinner I took an hour's nap and then went out to sit by the pool. I find myself sitting at poolside now with the not so disturbed residents, rather than under the balcony with the sicker ones as I did at first.

Barbara is manic tonight — walking continuously, singing, dancing, strutting, flirting. She's a show. The cool, pleasant evening has attracted a large number of people to sit at ease in the patio.

At 8 P.M. we watched the Olympics on television. I was reminded that at the hospital our looking at the all-star basketball game was interrupted by the scheduled movie call. Here, the choice is ours; the options remain open. B Home may not be a genuine path toward getting into the community, but it's a freer place than the schedule-bound mental institution.

To bed, writing "letters" until after 10 P.M. I've finished nearly a thousand pages of light reading since coming here. A book is a handy prop. It not only fills time and takes one away vicariously; it also tends to make one socially invisible while seated in the midst of people who are interacting with one another, and, furthermore, the margins provide a convenient place for note-taking.

August 29

When I got back for the recreation center activity schedule to begin at 3 P.M., I was told that people had gone to the beach instead, that the occupational therapy shop was closed, and that there would be no trip to Rustic Canyon as scheduled. I had heard no earlier announcement of the change in schedule. Disappointing. It is rumored that Leon wants to separate Kary and Beth. It is rumored that Beth has learned to hallucinate from Kary.

Bunny and Mary and quite a few residents were in the pool this afternoon. Mary invited me to join them, and I did. We played ball for a while; then they decided to play a game putting the two recreation therapists on the shoulders of two male residents — a version of "king of the hill." I wandered away. Another resident was holding Bobby up, teaching him to swim in the pool. Someone remarked that Bobby had a good buddy.

Our sheets were not changed nor were our beds made today. I wonder why. An oversight? The same thing has happened several times this week.

There has been no preferred menu slip in the box since mine was taken out on Saturday.

At 4:30 Leon announced that a group would be coming to entertain us at 7 P.M. He didn't know specifically what they would do, but he asked us to wait and see. Many of us did. I played bridge, waited, made a phone call, then waited some more. At 7:30 the entertainers arrived. What a farce! They were engaged in entertaining themselves, not us. For thirty or forty minutes they played the piano and sang for one another.

The leaders of the group were middle-aged females of the show-biz type. The group came from the ward of a local psychiatric hospital. Tonight Barbara was manic and hyperactive again. The visitors endured some of her loud off-key singing and her other attention-seeking activities, but they wanted attention, too. Finally, one leader put Barbara in her place (apparently with enjoyment; she said the right "professional" things, such as "I like you" and "I'm willing to notice you," but she radiated bitchiness at the same time). I don't know exactly what Barbara did to provoke the clash that she'd been working toward all evening. She cried and told the visitors to stay away from her. She would be going back to the hospital because they had upset her so much, she sobbed. Later Barbara dropped a Coke bottle on the cement. Glass was flying. It was the type of encounter in which sick people sicken one another. I learned later from Helen that Barbara jumped into the pool with her clothes on, ran around nude, and fled when they were about to take her back to the hospital. (These events occurred after I had gone to bed.)

At first the visitors played secular tunes on the piano, but later turned to hymns. By this time the B Home residents weren't paying much attention to the entertainers. Some watched the Olympics on TV while others chatted. I played Ping-Pong. Most of the residents recognized that the visitors were there to entertain themselves and so ignored them, though one resident did photograph a member of the group as he played the piano. Much later we learned that the group had come to B Home primarily to use our music room. It had been a gross mistake for the authorities to present the visitors as coming to entertain us.

The owners of B Home dropped in with two other well-dressed couples. They went into the office. In a few minutes the three ladies came out on the balcony. Mrs. B was pointing out various residents and discussing their disorders with her friends in a rather sympathetic way. Karl and Leon seemed to become quite visible after their boss arrived.

It was a confusing and upsetting evening for David Kent. He senses the undercurrent of disorganization and anger and he wants to hide from it in his room. Yet he needs to be with people, especially now that he sees less opportunity to be with people after his approaching change of residence. Kent will live alone.

Several friends have asked me if I'll stay another month. I've told them it's impossible. There's immediate stardom associated with leaving, but there are the beginnings of disengagement, too. No use getting deeply involved with someone whom you probably will never see again after Sunday.

August 30

Kary was taken to the hospital late last night because she was hallucinating. Barbara had run away so that she wouldn't be taken back to the hospital, too. She returned this morning, however, and seemed a bit more settled. Kary's absence stirred genuine concern among some residents. Sherry planned to visit her, taking along an enormous stuffed lion as a gift.

Wally, who had left B Home again to try life on his own, was already back. I asked about his decision to return. He explained that welfare benefits were cut down when he left the board-and-care home. Although this procedure is routine, he regarded the reduction as a punishment, an indication that the government prefers to have us stay here. The other factor was loneliness. As he put it, "You start talking to strangers in the park, and they have other people to talk to and other things to talk about."

After lunch I found Leon by the truck with a resident who was asking for a ride in the bus. Leon didn't want to take him along and didn't want to tell him where he was going (except to say it wasn't where the resident wanted to go). Leon was more than firm; he was almost arrogant. When I asked about the day's activities Leon quickly changed his demeanor; he became reasonable and even walked a few steps my way in order to hear better. He seems to respond to pushiness with his own pushiness and with a display of power, but he tends to react to softness in a more paternal way.

Leon told me that Mary isn't here today (I'd learned that earlier from Paul) and that no activities had been planned. There was no public announcement of this change, no effort to tell us why Mary was gone, no effort to substitute another activity — nothing. We are to accept gratefully what management throws to us (sometimes ill planned and ineptly carried out at minimal expense) and then wait for the next dole. It's dehumanizing and frustrating.

At poolside a resident reminded another that it was already 4:15. He had better get out of the pool and get ready for dinner. This incident is an example of Parkinson's first law in operation: when there is plenty of time we tend to fill it with an activity that could be done much more quickly. Dinner begins at 5 P.M.

Ruby, the black cook, was praising the same resident for going swimming (his first time today) and for shaving off his beard. "You look good. Getting out is good for you." This kind of folk therapy can be very effective. Ruby is a mothering type and rather playful. Every day she participates in a ritual exchange. When asked "What's for lunch [or dinner]?" she replies, "Food." "What kind of food?" "The kind peoples eat." What food we're going to have is not a well-kept secret; today I knew all three meals before we ate. Usually, however, the information comes from overheard conversations or from residents who help out in the kitchen, rather than from Ruby. The official policy of secrecy is maintained because some residents don't show up for a meal if they hear that something unappetizing, or something they don't like, is on the menu.

The housekeepers were changing our linen as I got back to our room. They acknowledged that they didn't get to our room yesterday. They had me empty the wastebasket and tell Paul that if he didn't pick up his clothes they were going to report him to the manager. Paul went directly to the room and picked up his belongings.

This evening there wasn't much to be done at the NOVA meeting, Dan said, and as he had another appointment we would have to make it quick. We didn't. The proceedings included questioning as to why some people pay $187 a month and others pay $193 a month and some pay even more. Another item on the agenda was arrangements for bathing and laundering for the few residents unable to do these things for themselves. Karl dropped in discreetly to remind us that Steve, our president, is leaving, that we'll miss him, and that he's welcome back anytime. After making the announcement Karl left quickly so that we wouldn't think he was spying on our meeting for the management. There was some debate as to whether a resident should stand up and state his name every time he spoke at a meeting. Wendell suggested that we do so and ultimately the formality was made optional, but not before he had noted that the longer our group remained in B Home the more we would take over the meeting and that then our organizer would "sit in the back." Wendell senses that Dan opposes his measure. He is also aware that Dan runs the meeting. It's no secret. But Dan does it without parading his superiority, using such phrases as "to restate what Steve has already said. . . ."

Talked with Adelaide and Rose at poolside. Adelaide has been here three years and says she can't leave for financial reasons. She and Rose confirm that welfare is cut back when one leaves a board-and-care home. I remarked that B Home seems to be a hospital ward in the community. They agreed, pointing out it's so expensive to keep patients in a hospital that administrators are anxious to push them out into board-and-care homes where the costs of housing them are lower.

Watched a fellow smuggling liquor into his third-floor room. Alcohol isn't permitted, but it turns up now and then.

August 31

Time is structured differently here from the way it is in the normal world. There are a few fixed anchor points (meals, bus schedule, canteen schedule, and the like) but lots of drifting, unspoken-for time in between. Jerry tries desperately to fill it with games and sleep. Many residents stuff the pillowcase of time with feathers of conversation. Some pace, others hallucinate. One man uses the television — almost "owns" it, it's so important to him — all day. But many of us to some degree have learned to relax and simply accept the passage of time, doing nothing. It's an art that, like any other, takes practice. If nothing else it extends life, perhaps not objectively, but subjectively.

I've lent $3.15 so far and got back $3.00. Not bad. I've refused loans to several people. It's easier to turn down people I don't know or people who already owe me money and to turn them down when I'm low on cash myself. (Is this natural defense against lending one reason that some soft touches seem to try to go through their money very quickly?) The same principles apply to cigarettes.

At breakfast someone asked Corky, "What's the matter?" "I'm nervous." "We're all nervous," said one resident. "Don't feel lonely," another said sympathetically.

I got back and played some pool. Joe was trying to borrow money from Shelley in order to eat out. "I can't eat in the dining hall." "Why not?" "I'm too nervous."

Housekeepers here are addressed by their first names by some of the residents and they know these residents' names, too. Informal relationships grow like vines on the trellis of formal social structures.

At suppertime I laid my pills on my napkin, displayed them, and then publicly threw them into the wastebasket in the TV room. No one said anything; there were no repercussions. Several times I've found pills that have fallen from my pocket on the floor of my room, but the maids don't seem to notice or report them.

After supper Leon announced that since Mary wasn't here (no reason given) there would be no bus to Stoner Park for the dance. Those who wanted to go could take public transportation. My feeling at the moment is that the management doesn't care whether or not we have something to fill up the long, empty hours.

Bridge and chess. Routine allows predictable escape from boredom.

Four of us — Mario, Barbara, Jose, and I — decided to go by bus to the dance. It looked like rain so I suggested we take my "friend's" car; he is on a trip and asked me to drive it occasionally to keep the battery charged. I told my companions to tell anyone who asked that we'd come by public bus, and they did so. Even at the end, when Bunny asked us separately if we wanted a ride home, we each responded that we would rather take "the bus." Sharing this secret and being B Home's representatives at the dance gave us a feeling of camaraderie. Barbara, despite her upset earlier this week, was perfectly normal; she became embarrassed when I mentioned her breaking a coke bottle the other evening.

At the park Bunny, the recreation therapist, turned off my query — "Have you ever gone out with a former mental patient?" — by showing me her ring and telling me how happy she was to have gotten it from her boyfriend. The query was handled tactfully. She went on to say that she had talked with Mary about me. They hoped I would make it on the outside. She volunteered her phone number and Mary's, suggesting that I call one of them if I needed to talk to someone. She also encouraged me to visit a local folk-dance hall that she frequents.

Knowing this was probably my last time at the park, Bunny spent most of the evening with me, asking me to help prepare the refreshments and clean up — more to keep her company than to work. I asked if she might get into trouble by giving me the phone numbers. "Staff members aren't supposed to have contact with us after working hours, are they?" I asked. "Don't think of me as a staff member," she replied. Difficult, but hopeful.

September 1

Up at 6 A.M. to write "letters." Breakfast at 7 A.M. The lights are switched out in the TV room a moment before the door to the dining room is opened. I wonder why this signal is given.

Helen learned the hard way that at our competitive table one grabs the milk for cereal when it's near or else there may be a long wait. Coffee and milk are poured first; sugar is taken later because there are two sugar dispensers on the table.

Leon chewed out Albert for telling people that he's allowed to eat pancakes at the diet table. Flo had believed the regular resident helper who in turn had believed Albert's statement that pancakes are part of his diet menu. But Leon would have none of it and Flo will be less credulous in the future.

After breakfast Helen and I talked. She has lost weight, as I have (5 lbs.), since coming here. She's recovering from an intestinal flu virus.

Talked with Rose at poolside. Rose does secretarial work for nothing (not even carfare) at the Jewish Community Center three afternoons a week. "It's something to do."

September 2

At breakfast I laid my pills on my napkin so Karl and the others could see them. Then I wadded up the napkin when Karl turned away. No comment. I push, but I meet no resistance.

I felt weak, so I lay down for about an hour after breakfast. No need to hurry things because there's lots of time; I took it easy and felt better. There are continual reminders that we have an unusual degree of freedom here.

Stu has what many call a "tranquilizer tan," a red-brown leather-like tan on his face and neck. He takes eleven tranquilizers a day. "I'd be dead right now if it weren't for tranquilizers," he says. No one here seems to think much of electroshock. Some people conceptually link shock treatments with electrocution.

Do we want people like Stu to move from board-and-care homes into the community? In many respects a board-and-care home is in itself a small community, a haven in which unwanted members of the larger society can be "stored." We mustn't assume that pushing people to move from these places will automatically enrich their lives. Here they find friends, acceptance, minimal competition, tolerance for idiosyncrasies. No wonder some of those who go out choose to return.

Herb banged on the door of the TV room and asked Karl for a fresh deck of cards. Karl gave me the keys and told me to run down to the storage room and bring up a new deck. He trusted me with all those keys.

How empty the canteen is tonight! One factor is the resident who is working there now. Since he is rather cold and unfriendly, people aren't likely to congregate there when he is on duty. Herb and Shelley, on the other hand, are more friendly, thus encouraging sociability.

Late at night someone was banging on a nearby door. "Let me in! Let me in!" At 4:30 in the morning Paul came in hallucinating, muttering, and sneezing; he began to jump in and out of bed. He asked me a question from his bed as if he knew I was awake. "Where's Jaime?" I replied that Jaime was probably home for the weekend. Again I was somewhat afraid to return to sleep, but I did after Paul quieted down, some forty-five minutes later. Paul plans to move into the annex with Jimmy on Monday. He lost the annex apartment he had earlier when he went "on vacation." He's anxious to go back. Poor Jimmy!

September 3

My last day at B Home. Got up and went outside by the pool. I wanted to look around and also to give people a chance to say good-bye. The last day is one of several vulnerable periods in which one can be confidently happy or can be crushed by slights from others. For me it turned out to be a disappointment and an anti-climax, for few people even knew that I was leaving.

After breakfast I asked Karl what I should do when I moved out that evening. He told me to turn in my key, pick up medication, and, if I wanted to, to leave a forwarding address in the event I got mail. His attitude was already one of disengagement. It seemed as if I had already gone. I, too, had begun disengaging a few days earlier. More and more of my thinking turned to what I would be doing after I had left. And I was spending more and more time away from B Home.

After lunch we played bridge. The fellows I played with all shook hands with me at the end and wished me luck. Jerry invited me to return for a visit. He seemed a bit more disheveled and disturbed than usual. It may have been because he was losing a valued game opponent. The rest of the afternoon, whenever I met my card-playing friends by chance, there was the expectable uncomfortable-ness of farewells already accomplished and of my being already socially gone.

It began to sprinkle. Something new to break up the routine. Bingo was played in the TV room today. Some residents thought there would be no bingo because it was too wet to sit by the pool, as if bingo had to be played at poolside or not at all.

I went in swimming despite the weather. Afterward a volunteer came by and asked to play checkers. He beat me in a few games, then I got Jerry, the gamester, to play him. Winning consistently, Jerry reclaimed B Home's honor.

I went back to my room. Interestingly, most of the males in B Home seem to do their socializing outside the rooms. One comes out to face society and retreats to one's room for privacy. Little inter-action seems to take place among roommates in the rooms. Although inviting guests to come inside does occur, it is not frequent.

As I waited for supper Mike told me he wished me luck; he said he could hardly wait till he was out of this place. We shook hands. This farewell was especially touching because Mike is a bitter, soured young man. His efforts to be thoughtful and open about missing someone are undoubtedly rare.

After supper I went to my room and brought down my suitcase. Bob saw me from his place at the table, smiled, and waved through the window, Rose told me good-bye and wished me good luck. Karl seemed distracted. He had to hurry back inside to finish giving out medications. We shook hands. I told him I hadn't been taking medications for the last few days but I'd better take along the rest in the event I would need them. No response except that he went to get my remaining Elavil. And I walked out the front door alone.

There is a need for an ending ceremony here (as there is a need at discharge from the mental hospital). The community should wish the departing person well, remind him that he's welcome to come back, and put a proper termination to his stay. Leaving alone is a sad thing and may be the kernel of the lonely vulnerability that leads to a suicidal act later. A lot depends upon whether one is pushing away from B Home or pulling toward something perceived to be better.

Looking back on my stay in this board-and-care home I can see why it is a haven, an ending point, for many residents. The rewards of life are simple but reasonable and the demands are very few. It is a sheltered world of acquaintance-peers with whom you need not compete. There is a benevolent authority to whom you can appeal for help in case of trouble — and hope for action. Within very broad limits (including financial and medical ones) one's freedom is unrestricted.

There are irritations, to be sure: fellow residents who create disturbances, the occasional insensitivity of managment, limitations on personal space, and an erratic schedule of activities. But these are relatively minor problems, provided one is able to lower his aspirations and confine his potential to fit the rewards offered by the system. It is not a bad place to live, but it is a terribly limiting one.

The setting for the next journal account was also B Home. Helen Sonier Sullivan, at that time a graduate student in clinical psychology at UCLA took on the identity of Helen Summers for the purposes of our study. The personal history of Helen Summers was created from Helen Sullivan's past, distortions of her past, profiles of suicidal persons seen at the Suicide Prevention Center, and from the fertile imaginations of our research staff. Her training included role playing and a brief period spent in the psychiatric ward from which she was to be discharged.

As noted earlier, the purpose of sending two experiential researchers into the same setting simultaneously was to enable us to distinguish the broader impact of the setting from David Kent's idiosyncratic perception of it. In this facility, as in most institutions, the pressures are sufficiently powerful to evoke similar responses from both researchers despite differences in background and personality.

HELEN SUMMERS'S B HOME JOURNAL

August 3

This afternoon Sharon, my social worker, took me out to the facility to look around and to be introduced as a prospective resident. My first impression was that B Home is a complex maze of areas and rooms with stairs connecting various places.

Once in the office, the woman at the desk put us in the charge of Don, the administrator. Don is a big black guy who jokes a lot and comes on in a kind of flirtatious way, but he seemed genuinely concerned to make me feel comfortable. Some of his cordiality, I felt, was based on a desire to "sell" the place (Sharon had told him that we were looking at several residences), but I think a great deal of it was real. We toured the patio, music room, library, TV room, dining room, canteen, and OT shop, and looked at several apartments.

With a few exceptions Don was careful to give me a sense of being included, of being a part of the decision as to what was going to happen to me. For example, he would physically include me in the circle when we stopped to talk, would address me personally, would ask me if I had any questions, and then he would wait to hear my answers. This approach is a very sensible one; it made me feel important, and I noticed the difference on the few occasions when he seemed to neglect me. Several times, when Sharon and Don took off ahead of me, laughing and joking (they had known each other before), I felt that I was very much in the way, as if I were a hapless third wheel.

Then Don started to tell Sharon about one of the girls living in B Home. He used the word "crazy" when describing her. I'm sure that I wouldn't have noticed if he hadn't become so embarrassed and started apologizing. Small as this incident was, it had a considerable effect in creating a distance between us, reinforcing our respective roles as patient and nonpatient.

There were subtle changes in voice pitch and vocabulary when Don spoke directly to me. I was speaking very quietly and he seemed to respond to that by speaking quietly in return. The softness of his voice was reassuring at a time when I was being bombarded on all sides by new impressions.

By the time we got back to his office I was totally confused as to how one place was connected to another; I couldn't remember the name of anyone I had met and the faces had all become a blur. At that point he wanted to know if I had any questions, but I couldn't think of a single thing to ask. I was grateful when he didn't push too hard, and Sharon filled in the gap by asking some questions of her own while I tried to collect myself. The brochure Don gave me was something to mull over in quiet by myself later. It would help to allay some of the anxiety about moving into a strange place.

August 8

I arrived at about three o'clock yesterday afternoon. Sharon came with me. The woman at the desk was professionally pleasant, but I got the impression that either I was unexpected or that it was inconvenient for me to arrive at that time. For the first ten minutes she spoke about me in the third person, talking with Sharon about forms, arrangements, and medication. I was already feeling rather anxious, and her attitude added an element of personal insignificance to the rest of what I was feeling. When she spoke to me, though, she was warm and welcoming, but her tone made the total message more confusing because she somehow retained that distracted air, period-ically calling on the intercom for someone — the call had something to do with me, I supposed. Then she had me sign a card, took my money, and gave me a key, explaining that the key was also to be used for opening the facility's back doors. At that juncture a man came into the office, introduced himself as Leon, and said he would show us to my room. He struck me as a somewhat brusque, perhaps overly efficient, sort of person. He asked if we had been to B Home before. When Sharon said we had, he proceeded straight to my apartment, although Sharon said I might need to be shown around again. In the room he showed me my bed, put his hands on my shoulders, told me that he hoped I would be happy there, and said I should come and see him if I wanted to talk about anything. Although he said nice things they didn't seem particularly genuine to me; he said them as if he was just doing his job. I had an un-explainable feeling of wanting to defend myself against this person.

What I am saying about Leon, however, may be very unfair. It is really too early to tell yet. After telling me that he would see me at dinner, Leon left.

There was a woman in the largest room in the apratment when we came in, but she didn't say anything to us. Leon didn't say anything to her either, and she was gone by the time he left.

My room is on the second floor, across from B Home's TV room. There are three rooms in this apartment, with four beds in all. The kitchen isn't equipped for cooking and the living room functions as a second bedroom. The rooms are fairly spacious. They have an un-crowded feeling, despite the usual feminine array of toilet articles and clothes. I sense a certain aura of impersonality about the place, as if there were minimal overlapping of the individuals living here. Each person has the right to half of whatever space is in his room. I found half of the bureau top, closet, and dresser drawers cleared for me.

I stayed in my room until dinner, feeling rather stranded. An-other woman entered and left her room a few times but she didn't say anything to me. My roommate didn't come in at all and from the few things scattered on her side of the room it was impossible to make any guesses about her age or anything else.

At five the other woman told me I could go to dinner if I wanted to. She asked me my name and told me that hers was Maureen. I was feeling quite apprehensive about facing so many new people at dinner and would have followed Maureen except that she bolted ahead.

I found the walk alone from my room to the dining room an interminable ordeal. I would never have left what I had already come to regard as the isolated security of my room except that I felt that I should find out what dinnertime was like. I felt extraordinarily grateful to Leon for appearing from nowhere to rescue me. He took me in and introduced me to the housefather. I still found it impos-sible to remember names or faces. When the housefather was gone I wasn't sure that I'd ever be able to recognize him again.

As the dining room was already full I went to the TV room to wait for the second serving of dinner. A young man with a sombrero, Sam, came over to talk to me. He asked a lot of questions. I had the impression that I was being hustled to a certain degree, but just as I was beginning to feel too invaded we were called into dinner.

I was struck by the almost total lack of conversation at our table.

People would ask or signal for what they wanted, eat silently, and then quickly leave.

The woman in charge of the serving — I think she might be the housemother — impressed me as an exceptionally warm and motherly person. She bustled around, mopping up spills, handing our food to us, clucking over people as if this "collection" were her family. Although I had never been introduced to her she seemed to know my name and made me feel very welcome.

After dinner I went to sit outside for a while. Although I hadn't noticed any social pressure to leave my room that afternoon, there was certainly more pressure to socialize once I got outside. Several other men besides Sam came over to talk to me. Soon I started feeling hassled and wanted to be alone. I said I was going upstairs, and I left. No explanation was necessary. In fact, I believe I could have said nothing and simply left.

I stayed in my room reading for the rest of the evening, partly because I really wanted to be alone and partly because I wanted to see if there would be any effort to bring me outside. No one said anything; I went to bed early.

At about 12:30 A.M. I was awakened by the sound of someone moving in the room. At about the same time I heard the sound of rushing water; a fire hydrant had burst outside my window. When I sat up a woman in her fifties was standing next to my bed looking out the window. I asked her what the noise was. She replied that "they" were trying to put out a fire. She said that a fire was burning up the whole world and Christ was being burned by fire and men were after her. She went on in this way for quite some time. Already feeling somewhat disoriented, I was frightened by her strange talking. I was an inexperienced resident who had just arrived and didn't know what to expect next. Although I kept trying to go back to sleep, I would periodically become aware of her presence and would start up to find her leaning over me, looking for a cigarette, eyeing the clock, or just staring at me. It's hard to describe the anxiety and the sheer terror I felt then. I wasn't thinking rationally. As time passed, when she wasn't standing over me she began to rummage through closets and drawers, taking things out, putting them back again. I don't think she sat down for more than five minutes. She certainly never lay down. At 4:30 A.M., giving up all hope to sleep, I got up and started to get dressed. With my contact lenses in I felt better able to face any crisis. I set about retrieving my possessions which this woman had scattered about the room. Meanwhile the woman who had come back into the room, told me her name was Margaret. She helped me find my things. At last I was beginning to think more rationally. We talked off and on for the next couple of hours while I crocheted. It occurred to me that Margaret might have been as unnerved by my presence as I was by hers. Although she continued to drift off into personal fantasies at times, she was quite coherent in other moments, even exhibiting a gentle caring for me. She was concerned that I might be crying when I was rubbing my eyes, touching my face, worrying about my breakfast, and so forth.

Actually, I found myself becoming quite fond of Margaret during those early morning hours. Still, I was aware of a persistent trembling that has continued through much of this day. Part of it is a result of lack of sleep, I know, but part of it comes from the intense terror I felt, however unfounded it may have been. It is a new place, the apartments are relatively isolated, and even the two people in the next room seem strange and distant.

This afternoon I sat in the TV room until dinner. It seems to be another good place for me to be left alone. There is virtually no interaction among patients except for routine bumming of cigarettes and swapping of ashtrays. Occasionally a comment was made about the television program, but it didn't seem to be addressed to anyone in particular.

The man sitting next to me introduced himself as Paul. He is a tall, serious-looking man, probably in his early forties. He works on a psychiatric hospital newspaper as part of an incentive program. Although he seemed very shy he offered the information that he had been at B Home for three years and told me that if I needed to know anything I could ask him. Aside from this exchange, everything else was about the same as yesterday — a solitary meal with everyone silent, eating as quickly as possible in order to get out. With its rush for position and a minimum of conversation, mealtime reminds me mostly of a hospital, right down to the man across from me putting his meat between two pieces of bread and carrying the sandwich out in a napkin.

Again I watched television for a while after dinner. There seems to be a hard-core viewer atmosphere about this room. There is also a ritual selection of programs, probably the same programs day after day.

More patients have begun to talk to me. More men than women, but I suppose that's because I'm a woman. The girls closer to my age seem to have an already well-established group. They appear to be considerably more outgoing than I feel.

I have the sense of a certain community spirit with individuals concerned about how I feel; they work at drawing me out. At the same time there is a noticeable respect for my past. Questions are fairly unobtrusive; beyond asking where I'm from no one has wanted to know much about me or how I got here. I'm still having trouble with names and faces. The residents introduce themselves gradually, rather than all at once as the staff did.

August 9

Last night when I went to my room a girl named Ann was there with Margaret. She said she was an outpatient at the hospital. She had known Margaret for several years and come home with her because Margaret had appeared rather disturbed during the day. Ann is an energetic, forthright person, and I found her enlisting my aid as one might ask an older child to help with a younger one. First she reinforced my potential for wellness, pointing out that I had been hospitalized for only a short time and that soon, like her, I would be ready to go outside, resume a normal life, and perhaps return to school. Then she drew on my own experience with illness to create some understanding of what Margaret must be going through. Not all of this talk was necessary at this point, because my feeling toward Margaret had changed with daybreak yesterday. Still, she had a very effective style of mobilizing resources.

Ann was concerned that Margaret was becoming more upset. She had come prepared to spend the night, if necessary. Evidently Margaret has been known to injure herself accidentally and has started a couple of fires, confirming my earlier fears. It also seems that Margaret is not always this way. I wonder why it was Ann who noticed the change rather than one of the staff members. It makes me think that one can readily achieve anonymity around here, and that is a dangerous possibility for a potentially suicidal patient.

When Margaret became difficult for even Ann to handle, the houseparents were consulted. They gave me the impression of being quite ill at ease with the situation. Flo, the housemother, made one attempt to talk to Margaret, but retreated when Margaret pushed her off. I like the houseparents, but as another resident I had a sudden feeling of insecurity. If I were upset and frightened I would want someone there stronger than I, someone who could take charge of my world and hold it together, not someone who would be frightened off. The houseparents went to call Don. Eventually Margaret was taken back to the hospital.

I can't be sure yet what the authority hierarchy is, but I suspect from this incident that Don is somewhere near the top and the houseparents are somewhere near the bottom, though their ineffectiveness may be partly owing to their newness and their relative unfamiliarity with B Home. Leon drives the bus. Although I don't know where he stands in the hierarchy, he may be important, for he speaks and carries himself with some authority. Also I've noticed that some of the residents treat him with deference.

Of course, there are the B's who own the place. I'm not sure how involved they are in actually running it. From what I've heard from several of the residents, however, I gather they are nice people who provide periodic social gatherings for the residents.

Finally, a man named Karl seems to have a lot to do with the daily operation of B Home. Although I personally don't have much contact with him I have the feeling that he knows everybody and everything that happens around here. He is a very practical, matter-of-fact person. He doesn't set himself apart from the residents as other staff members do. If he likes the program on TV he is likely to sit down and watch it. For all his casual purposefulness, he is probably the key person to the successful running of B Home.

Don came over to talk to me after dinner. I had not seen him since my visit on Friday. He wanted to know how I was getting along. He seemed especially concerned about how I was feeling after the Margaret episode. I had the feeling that he was watching me very carefully to see whether or not I was disturbed. Although he mentioned that he doesn't get a chance to see much of me because he works days, he did say that he had seen me leave early the day before. I had conflicting feelings about this remark: it was reassuring to have someone keeping an eye on me and watching out for me, yet it was also a subtle reminder that my comings and goings are under scrutiny. At least they are publicly visible should anyone happen to be watching.

I watched people playing billiards in the canteen tonight. It was the first time I had wandered in there. Always before when I had glanced in to the room the people there seemed so comfortable there that I felt out of place and slightly more depressed.

Already formed groups, laughing and playing together, are hard for the new resident. Although it was fun to watch for a while, I soon felt even more alone. I could deal much more easily with individuals.

There are feuds here, but for the most part they are limited to low rumblings and mutterings when opposing factions meet. Thus far I've observed the tendency to argument mostly in the television lounge, where somebody enters and somebody else (Sam, for instance) sinks into his chair and starts muttering under his breath.

August 10

At dinner tonight I was sitting next to Rosa, one of my roommates. She is a quiet, warm, motherly little woman. She introduced me to her friend Arline who was sitting on the other side of her. When Karl came to our table to pass out medication, Arline said that the male residents would probably go wild if they didn't have their pills. There was a sharp sense of superiority in her voice. I wondered if dependence on pills is another status distinction here, in addition to those who work versus those who don't and the young versus the old. At that point Rosa got her pill, too. I wondered how she felt after that comment from friend.

I am aware of how basically neat and uncluttered the home is. Although I haven't noticed any directives to this effect, there seems to be a common effort toward keeping the place clean, using the ash cans, placing stray Coke bottles in the rack, and the like. Perhaps this behavior reflects an unspoken pride in the appearance of one's "home." The absence of any stray personal possessions may represent a fear of theft. My own experience hasn't supported that worry, however, for I accidentally left a sweater in the TV room one night and found it there the next day on my way to dinner.

I had planned to go to the dance tonight to see what it was like, but I didn't go because I had no information on the details, such as where to meet and when. Although just about everybody — including myself — seems to know about the existence of activities, there is no specific procedure for informing people about the mechanics involved in participating.

At 9:15 P.M. the area is very quiet. Most of the people seem to have gone to the dance or to bed. Six or seven men are in the TV room watching the fight. There is a small group of young girls down at the end of the pool.

August 11

Last night after supper I went up to "my" patio table in the corner of the second-floor porch and watched the people on the patio below. I found myself getting very depressed. I think one of the things that triggered my depression was the despair accompanying a feeling of closeness to some of the people here. I was thinking especially of Alvin, a little old man I had talked to before dinner. He looks as if he had had a stroke, for he has little control over his facial muscles, speech is difficult for him, and he drools. His gait also seems to be affected. He has some interesting things to say, but people shy away from him just because he is difficult to understand. I found myself worrying about the narrowness of his life. He is virtually alone in the midst of all these people. What does he have to look forward to?

I hate the presumptuousness of that kind of thinking, as if I could judge the worthiness of someone else's life or assess the happiness or unhappiness of other people. Still, I can't help it. The more I see and talk to people, the worse I feel.

Helen, the researcher, is depressed about the hopelessness of this type of institution. What each one of these people needs — what we all need — is to have at least one other person really love and care for us. That seems impossible here. I am convinced that the staff members here see their roles as more than mere jobs. There is genuine feeling between them and many of the residents. But there are not enough of them, and there never will be.

Helen Summers has been coming out of her initial depression and anxiety enough to notice a great deal more of what is happening around her. What she notices, however, is groups of interconnected people who present a sharp contrast to her own aloneness. Hence, more depression. Also, she is becoming more aware of the dead-end atmosphere in the place, and that is frightening.

Even if you accept the proposition that some of the people here have everything they want and are quite happy (which, I think, is probably true), Helen Summers and Helen Sonier have in common the knowledge that they have both experienced other ways of life and have found them more fulfilling, even though disappointing at times. They still have places to go. The recognition that most of the people here are already at the end of the road is upsetting. So far, I have heard only two people talk vaguely about leaving. Few people have asked me how long I plan to stay (implying that I will be leaving). Rather, the question is, "Do you think you're going to like it here?"

At 9:45 P.M. I am writing in the bathroom because that's the only place I can have a light without disturbing anyone.

I have been lying in bed for about an hour now, feeling like a prisoner and getting more and more desperate about it. I can't sleep because there is a band playing rock music across the street, someone is banging on the floor above us, and there is an unusually large number of racing engines down in the street tonight. I don't think there are many experiences worse than being unable to sleep and being unable to move around or read or do anything at all about it.

I doubt very much that my sleeplessness is unique here. Yet, so far as I can see, there isn't much to be done about it. I can't turn on my light or I'll disturb my roommate; the living room is another bedroom so turning on a light there is out of the question, too. The same applies to the kitchen, which is not separated at all from the living room-bedroom. The TV room (when it is open) is dimly lit. The library-music room seems to have been taken over by jazz enthusiasts, whose music is too loud to permit one to read there comfortably. The canteen is now closed, and the patio is too chilly and too poorly lit. Walking alone at night on the street doesn't seem to be a particularly good idea either. Complain . . . complain . . . complain.

This afternoon there must have been at least eight men sitting in chairs at the entrance stairwell, smoking and listening to a radio one of them had. This place reminds me of a back ward in a state mental hospital. The light is cold, the walls are bleak, the chairs are lined up against the wall, and scattered cans contain smoldering cigarette butts. The men who sit there rarely go outside.

While I was sitting by the pool crocheting Leon came by, asked me what I was making, and complimented me on it. I felt mildly annoyed with him because he didn't wait to hear my answer. Perhaps he didn't expect me to answer. I felt like a faceless blob on the chair. Of all the staff, I feel most distant from Leon. His stride has a swagger; his voice is loud and jarring. His mannerisms remind me that he has real power over my life.

Don came over and asked to see me. I asked if he wanted to see me at that moment and he said only if it was convenient for me. It was an incredibly nice thing to hear. My time was important to someone. When I got up to the office Don told me to pack up my things. I had an instant of gripping paranoia — perhaps I had been discovered! But he went on to inform me that he was moving me into another apartment so that I would have a roommate. Don asked if the move was all right with me.

Although I can appreciate the necessity of switching people around, the move gives me a sense of disruption, even though I have been here only a few days. The feeling of being uprooted may be magnified for a person whose room has been and probably will continue to be his only home for some time. Perhaps room changes contribute to the absence of strong ties between most roommates and to the relative absence of efforts to personalize one's room. Don't get too involved; you might be taken away.

Tonight, watching TV after dinner, I became aware that I've been accepted into the B Home community. I'm not a new resident any longer. Maureen asked to borrow the key to our room. When I explained that Don had moved me and I no longer had a key, she said that she was sorry I was gone, that I had been a good roommate. It was the first reaching out I had experienced from her and it made me feel accepted. Coming from a woman it was especially important. Thus far, most of my interactions here have been with men; the women have kept a wary distance. That's what it's all about here — residents dealing with one another. Since nearly all my major contacts are with the other residents, it is ultimately they who make me feel better or worse.

This morning, after washing clothes, I went to the doughnut shop down the street for a cup of coffee and a paper. On my return Leon came stalking by and, in his usual brusque and too hearty manner, teased me about buying outside coffee. Still somewhat unsteady and unsure of myself, I find myself feeling more stupid and awkward and graceless each time I interact with him. I don't think my reaction is idiosyncratic because I've seen others wince under his heaviness, and a few scurry away rather than confront him. I'm not capable of the quick retort his wit seems to demand, and I don't feel helped by the cheery, buck-up attitude he so readily assumes.

A group left for Disneyland with an air of flurry and activity. After they left I became aware of a distinct letdown feeling among those of us who were left behind, a settling down into the humdrum routine of another weekend. I don't know all the reasons people had for not going, but I suspect that the five-dollar entry fee was a hindrance to some.

August 13

This morning Karl called someone for his medication. Seeing the patient across the patio, Karl came down the steps joking that he would come halfway. To come halfway is, both literally and figuratively, characteristic of Karl. Thus he communicates his valuing of residents as persons.

I watched a man make the rounds of the patio emptying ash cans. More and more I am aware of various inconspicuous housekeeping tasks that seem, for the most part, to be taken care of by residents.

Rosa and Maureen stopped by my table to talk. After a time I learned that they were concerned and hurt that I might have asked to be moved out of their apartment. I assured them that I had had nothing to do with it. They seemed relieved. Until then I felt that they didn't care one way or the other that I was in the room. Perhaps it was just part of the wariness I'd observed, especially among women, waiting for the intruder to prove herself.

At lunch I felt uncomfortable when Karl came to our table to hand out medication. My reaction struck me as odd because I really like Karl, especially his style of interacting with residents. While I was eating, I suddenly realized what the problem was: Karl doesn't treat me like a patient as the rest of the staff does. I was suspicious that he might have found out about me. Then I realized that he doesn't treat me like a patient because he doesn't treat any of the residents that way. This realization makes me feel a lot easier.

After lunch I spent some time sitting outside crocheting. Flo came over to see what I was making and made a big deal about it. Usually I felt safe and secure under her intense mothering, but today I was vaguely resentful of her praise. I expected her to look at what I was doing, remark that it was a nice job, and let it go at that. Her extravagant reaction was offensive. It was as if she was surprised that I could be capable of doing such a nice piece of work. Certainly, I was overreacting. Yet I felt like retorting that former mental patients can be as creative and skillful as anyone else.

On my way to bed I saw Karen crying. She was led from her room by Leon who was trying to reassure her. Maureen and her friend were sitting at my table, and I went up to ask them what was happening. They said Karen was merely upset about something, nothing new. I've already developed the instinct that sent me to another resident for information, rather than to the staff.

This afternoon I decided that I couldn't stand the usual total inactivity. I've begun to feel like a caged animal, restless, pacing. I've been used to a much more active life. It has been pleasant having everything done for me, but the experience has begun to pall. Perhaps that is why so many people here have invented a thousand routines for themselves. Anyway, I've started to participate, beginning with Ping-Pong and pool. Actually, I enjoy the games, though I worry about becoming too conspicuous. Just as there is the sensitivity among residents for the moment when you want to be left alone, there seems to be an equal awareness of the moment when you are ready to start engaging in life again. Any number of people seemed to be ready to teach me and help me to have fun.

August 14

More than any other area, the canteen is constantly changing with people coming and going, having fun in different ways. More and more I find myself (like many others) gravitating to the canteen, enjoying the distraction in a kind of vicarious way. Yet, in the end the vicariousness is itself a problem, and realization of that fact can make one depressed. At this point the most satisfied people here seem to be the ones who have found a niche in which they can do something — such as working in the kitchen, emptying ash cans, or, as in Georgia's case, working her own garden — rather than always having things done for them.

Talked to David Kent for a few moments. Perhaps we will be able to talk occasionally without attracting too much attention.

Afterward, I wandered around. Same people in the same places. Same program on television. In only one week the novelty has worn off and an established routine has emerged. Amazing and more than a little depressing.

Earlier in the evening I watched an interesting custom. Certain people were sent by other residents to get coffee for them. Evidently there are those who go and those who send. I suspect this hierarchy has an economic foundation, because those who run the errands seem to receive a few coins for their trouble or are allowed to get something for themselves.

I noticed again the lovely bunch of flowers that Georgia picked yesterday and arranged in a Coke bottle on our dresser. It's the first decorator touch I've noticed in either of the apartments in which I've lived. Quick glimpses into the younger girls' apartments suggest that they do more in the way of prettying up their rooms than the older women, whose rooms are rather barren, arranged in a utilitarian sort of way, and devoid of domestic touches. I'm not sure whether apathy in this respect reflects the transient nature of residency here, lack of money for frills, or just a general giving up and not caring anymore. Perhaps it is a combination of all these factors. Since many of the women here have had homes and families of their own in the past, they must not always have been so uncaring.

August 15

My depression seems to be giving way to a schizophrenic state in which I'm three different people. I'm finding it difficult to slip in and out of three identities in a single day. I think the ex-patient identity is the most persistent. Sometimes I find it intruding un-expectedly when I try to do something on the outside. Even when it doesn't surface obviously, it stays in the background of my aware-ness so that I find myself distracted to some degree when I try to do something else.

I've lost at least five pounds this first week. I was so down when I came here that I ate almost nothing for four days. My anxiety seemed to serve as an appetite depressant. Although I often left my plate of food virtually untouched, there was no reaction from the staff. With the exception of the loaf of bread always on the table, there is none of the heavy concentration of starch so often associated with institutional cooking. Residents seem quite satisfied with the food. I haven't heard the traditional griping common to patients in hospitals and students in dormitories.

August 16

Last night there was a fight on the patio before dinner. I think it was triggered by the man who had been yelling obscenities out by the stairs earlier. Karl quickly broke up the fight. For the most part arguments here seem to be confined to verbal exchanges, and the physical expression of hostility is unusual. Most of us here are afraid of our strong emotions. We walk away rather than remain in a situation where they might emerge.

At the end of a meal I would enjoy lingering over a cup of coffee, perhaps with a cigarette. But smoking is not allowed in the dining room. When I decided that the continual mild stomachache I suffered during the first week might be caused by eating too fast, I made myself slow down. Eight minutes after I started I was alone at the table and someone was clearing the plates away. There is relentless pressure to bolt my food and flee.

At dinner today I made a pleasant discovery. I was sitting across from a man named Paul who customarily walks around the patio, talking to himself or to the bushes. After chatting with him for a while I realized that he talks to himself when other people don't talk to him, and that happens fairly often because he is shy about initiating conversations. One problem here is that those who cannot or will not reach out to others may find their existence terribly lonely. If you look around the patio carefully, even when it seems to be bright and gay, you will see many isolated, lonely-looking people.

While we were in the canteen Brook, Karen, and Shelly came in to play. For a while there was a lot of loud gaiety. Then Brook began a vicious attack on several of the older men who had come in. She made disagreeable comments about their behavior, their clothes, and their appearance. This appalling act of cruelty made the others nervous and uncomfortable, but no one made a move to go to the defense of her victims. I, too, felt bound by some unspoken code that prohibited interfering. I was too upset and angry to remain in the canteen. The influence residents have on one another can be constructive or destructive. The largely unchanneled potential for helping one another can be perverted to a tendency to tear one another apart.

Rosa had a bad toothache and swollen face last week and had finally been able to go to a dentist. Although the pain had temporarily subsided, the tooth was abscessed and should come out. Since Rosa's welfare medical stamps have not been arriving regularly, her family dentist of twelve years will not pull out the tooth. He wants to get the stamps first. What is striking is Rosa's unquestioning attitude about the affair. For her, as well as for so many others here, control over her money and over many other details of her life is invested in a distant bureaucracy. It never occurs to her that she has the right or the ability to question or influence this agency. Rosa's immediate contact with the welfare people at this time is a worker named Miriam. Rosa is afraid to bother Miriam too often, that is, more than once a month when the check hasn't arrived. Miriam, on the other hand, doesn't involve Rosa at all in the process by which her money will come, nor does she let Rosa know what's happening when it's late. All my friend knows is that she has no money, no stickers, and a tooth that is disintegrating with agonizing spasms of pain.

August 17

Yesterday morning I met Minnie, the cleaning lady. She took her coffee break so we could talk for a while. She is a warm sort of person with a fairly deep involvement in the lives of many of the residents. I imagine that for some residents she is an unheralded but important source of interaction.

August 18

Last night I went to the dance at Stoner Park. I talked Rosa into going. (It wasn't hard to persuade her.) We were the only women on the bus, besides Mary, and she doesn't count because she's staff.

There is a definite sense that if you want to go anywhere you have to be fast in order to get to the bus first. Since the facility's bus holds only fourteen or fifteen people, it is necessary to rush aboard. The limited space arouses competition and rivalry, rather than co-operation, when we go on outings. The bus filled up quickly after we got on. One man, dressed impeccably in honor of the occasion, was left standing by the garage as we pulled out. I was surprised at the coldness of those on the bus toward the ones left behind. When a resident dared to express his regret that a fellow was to be left at home, Mary replied sarcastically, "If you want to get out and give him your seat, go right ahead." Her tone ridiculed and mocked him. "After all, I take the first ones who get here and I'm certainly not going to make two trips!"

The dance itself was interesting. When we got off the bus we were herded along by several young people, presumably volunteers. They seemed quite enthusiastic, but they confused us because some of them urged us upstairs to a dance hall while others pressed us toward a volleyball court. Rosa and I allowed ourselves to be maneuvered upstairs. The few people in the hall when we got there were sitting singly on benches placed against the walls. At one end of the room music blared from a record player. At the opposite end long tables covered with paper contained painting materials. A few people came over to introduce themselves, but after the introductions were over there were uncomfortable gaps of silence because there were not enough people yet for the party to become lively. I was reminded, in a nightmarish way, of dances I attended when I was in seventh grade. Rosa and I escaped downstairs to watch the others play volleyball.

The players all seemed to be having a good time. Each team contained a mix of good and bad players, and everyone was included in the play. While we were watching the game a young man named Tom who came over to talk with us, kept trying to get me to go for coffee with him. His approach cut through the layers of sparring that usually take place when men and women are first getting to know one another. He assumed that we were both there for the same reason — to find someone to be with. When it began to get dark everyone went upstairs for the dance. Tom had since wandered off in search of more cooperative company. There was a lot of mingling between residents and volunteers. Both groups seemed to know most of the other people who came on a regular basis.

One of the volunteers came over to tell Jerry that Carol, a volunteer with whom he usually danced, was not there because she had to go to a funeral. The volunteer's effort was especially thoughtful because Jerry, who had dressed up hours before the dance in anticipation, had told us about Carol and might have been embarrassed by her unexplained absence. A lot of people danced, although others (like David Kent) painted on the long tables or sat in small groups and talked. All in all, the dance was a successful, important occasion.

While we residents waited for Mary to unlock the bus door there was speculation about how long she would make us wait, in comparison with other occasions. I don't think the staff members are aware of how much we observe and talk about them. They seem to think that we pick up only that part of a communication which they direct to us. They are wrong. We also understand facial expressions, gestures, pauses, and the like, as well as remarks made in our presence but not intended for us.

Tonight Don was standing next to me in the canteen for quite a while, but he didn't notice me. I'm convinced that if I am quiet and don't cause any particular trouble, I simply disappear into a wall. It occurred to me that I could make a fuss in order to get some attention, but that course of action doesn't fit into the nature of either Helen Summers or Helen Sonier. I'm beginning to understand, though why a resident might be driven to such an extreme.

Weekend evenings don't differ from any other evenings here.

Ed asked me to be his girl friend the first time we met. Sam had assured me early on that I would get well if I would learn to "be" with men. I've heard some rumors linking Bill and me. In this milieu, if you play two Ping-Pong games together you are practically engaged. At this point it seems best to move around, dividing my time among many people and never going out with anyone, even for coffee.

Tonight I also decided to try to break the television system. So at eight o'clock I went into the TV room and announced my wish to watch a particular program at nine o'clock. The people there agreed and I went out. When I returned, however, there were only a few people left and Joe would not allow the channel to be changed. There could be no discussion of the next program to be watched. Joe is recognized by everyone, including me, as the unofficial authority in the TV room. I stamped out, on the verge of a tantrum for the second time this evening.

August 19

A feeling of slowness is an established part of the weekend routine. It's common to hear such comments as "the weekend to get through," "such a long day," and "nothing to do." We have to accept the standard evening routine of sitting in the patio, wandering over to the canteen, coming back to the pool, checking out the TV, going to our rooms, trying the patio again, and so on. It is at such a time, when the weekend monotony sets in, that the waiting for visits and telephone calls becomes particularly noticeable. Today I heard some of the others kidding Larry and Joe for sleeping so late. But, as Joe put it, "What else is there to do?"

I am struck by the relative unproductiveness of so many of the members of this particular social system. Over time, nonproductivity tends to lower the activity and motivation levels, thus producing a self-perpetuating cycle. I notice that my own motivation to do anything at all is severely reduced. It's all I can do to establish minor routines to keep myself moving. People are always willing to be entertained, yet they are never totally satisfied because entertainment cannot continue for twenty-four hours a day. And when it ends the void returns.

August 20

I wandered around today, essentially just waiting for something — lunch, *anything* — to happen.

When it was time to play bingo, Leon assigned the job of calling out the numbers to a resident named Clint. From his reaction it was obvious that this job is something of a privilege. He was doing a miserable job of it, however, and soon, along with the others around me, I found myself muttering under my breath at his inefficiency. Suddenly, suffering an epileptic seizure, he fell over. Most of those in the room were frozen by the incident; a few shouted out suggestions to no one in particular. Someone called to Leon who came immediately. Although at one point I heard David Kent say something to Leon about protecting Clint's arms from getting burned on the hot cement, it seemed to me that Leon handled everything quite well, dispersing people without yelling at them, and generally tending to Clint until the ambulance arrived. Most people made the transition from intense irritation with Clint one minute to considerable concern for him the next. I am aware that the more cooped up I feel, the less tolerant and more easily irritated I tend to be. Anyway, I felt myself getting upset partly because this incident reminded me of another that occurred a long time ago. I decided to go for a walk, but as I passed the telephone booth by the back door of B Home a traffic sign fell over and, narrowly missing my head, landed on my foot. It was the last straw. With the shock and the pain, I broke down and started to cry hysterically as I ran to my room. People were kind, trying to find out what was wrong and offering their help. I don't remember much. I wasn't terribly rational at that point. By the time I had soaked my foot in the tub for a while, I was back together again. Several people had suggested that I go to Leon. He would know what to do.

What tremendous responsibilities Leon and the other staff members have! From minor problems (such as finding Howard's radio or breaking up a squabble at dinner or getting medical care for an injured toe) to major crises (such as Clint's seizure), we depended on the staff for solutions. Of course, it would be better all around if the staff would encourage residents to take more responsibility for their own affairs.

The aftereffects of Clint's seizure remained for a time. In the canteen there was talk about seizures, who had them, how recently, and so on. Underneath it all was the question: since it happened to him, could it also happen to me? to him? to her? The tension in the air was evidenced by several flare-ups at dinner. Perhaps a bit on edge himself, Leon came down hard on the participants in both incidents.

After dinner I talked to a man named Wendell. In the course of the conversation he asked me how old I was. He told me he was twenty-four when he got sick, and that had been twenty-two years ago. He said that I had a long time ahead of me. Then, a little less than optimistically, he remarked that he hoped I would have better luck than he had. I found this "preview" of my future to be tremendously depressing.

August 22

I came back from the VA early today in order to go to the Rustic Canyon Recreation Center. As late as 3:00 P.M., however, Mary and the others continued to splash around in the pool, making no move to get out and get dry. I felt cheated and disappointed because I had been looking forward to going there. As far as I could determine there was no explanation or announcement that the outing had been canceled.

After dinner I talked to Warren for some time. He will leave tomorrow to take a private room in Santa Monica, and he's feeling rather anxious about the prospect. He dwells on the times he tried to go out on his own before and failed. I think his own forebodings may make him fail again. It was clear, too, that the other people who stopped to talk with us a few moments didn't hold much hope that he would make a go of it on the outside, at least not for a long time. Their feelings about Warren's chances were communicated in subtle ways, but they may be crucially related to his success or failure. There doesn't seem to be any kind of structured send-off here for people leaving the home. Perhaps something of the kind is needed. Warren seemed to be in a sort of limbo, both being here and yet already gone at the same time. He seemed to be trying desperately to elicit some reaction from us concerning his leaving.

August 24

Don called out to me from the pool that he had heard I would be leaving. I felt uncomfortable yelling across the patio so I went downstairs to talk with him. He asked what I planned to do. I told him that I was going back to school and needed to live closer to school, probably in a dorm. Don said that he was very happy for me and told me that I should feel free to come and talk to him whenever I wanted to or needed something. He said that I was always welcome to come back to visit the home and use the pool. He noted that some residents who left two or three years ago still come back regularly. He also said that dorms could sometimes be very lonely places, especially on weekends, and that if I liked I could call and arrange to spend a few days at B Home. He expressed regret at not getting to know me better, but said that I was so shy — nice, but shy. He said some very good things to me. Unfortunately, I heard beautiful speeches when I came here and as I was about to leave, but very little in between.

Don's shouting to me on the balcony had evidently alerted the whole place that I would be leaving. Barbara came over to ask why I was going. She didn't want me to go. Don told her that I had to leave when I was ready to get on with my life, an explanation she seemed to accept. She was pleased to learn I wouldn't be leaving the next day. Her response to my departure surprised me because, although we share the same suite and have talked a few times, we really haven't been all that close. Perhaps Barbara is still unsure of herself here. She still talks about going back to the hospital. Maybe any kind of change is unsettling for her.

August 25

I still feel unsettled and agitated at my inability to sort out the feelings associated with leaving. My reluctance to leave stems to some degree from the relative involvement I've achieved this last week. Yet, though I may be more involved than David Kent, I'm certainly not as caught up in relationships as some of the other residents are. I wonder about those for whom this place has been "home" for several years, about those who, like Sandy, have adopted family substitutes. I wonder if the sense of familiarity, security, and sureness might not outweigh the inconvenience of living here, making it difficult to leave.

Also, while I know I can make it on the outside, I am aware of a tiny scared feeling within me. If I let myself dwell on the feeling I realize that it takes strength to live outside, but it really does not require that much strength to live here. Here we exist like the small boy who can practice flexing his muscles, but if something really "heavy" comes along he has his father by his side to give him a hand.

Living outside requires one to make choices, to reach decisions, and to take the initiative. Interpersonal relationships here are less demanding. Although I interact on several different levels with different people here, I have entered into an unspoken contract by which we agree to leave large portions of ourselves unexplored.

Last night as I sat on the patio with Herb and others, John came by and started his usual verbal dive-bombing routine. "Hi, what's your name? Pretty — oh, hi there — pretty." We asked him if he wanted to join us and he sat down and began his usual game of "Are you — — — ?" filling in the blank with a variety of famous names. For the most part, people responded by laughing, not derisively, but rather condescendingly. This reaction merely seemed to stimulate John to continue. I decided to try something different. So I turned to him, "John, I think you've just been putting us all on. You're making fun of all of us." The others acted as if I was out of my mind, but John gave me a strange look of acknowledgment and proceeded to fill the next few minutes with the most coherent, fluid conversation I had ever heard from him. His new self lasted until Chris, a new, young resident, came and sat down with us. At best Chris is unnerving. Within the space of five minutes he introduced himself fifteen times. Having been assured that we remembered his name, he moved from person to person, staring at each for two or three minutes at a time, exhibiting general dis-ease in his new surroundings. Finally he sat down and, without asking, started to drink from John's bottle of Coke. John became angry, but, instead of effectively directing his anger at Chris, he began to mutter rapidly to himself and took off with his strange gait. Chris, apparently unperturbed, took that initial long sip and then didn't touch the bottle again. He looked satisfied, as if his task had been completed. Chris impresses me as a spoiled child who appropriates everything within his grasp, someone who seeks attention by doing outrageous things.

Tonight as I was leaving the canteen Jerry suddenly leaned over and kissed me. I felt both embarrassed and somewhat taken aback since I couldn't be sure of exactly what lay behind that gesture.

Barbara has been quite agitated tonight. She talks about wanting to go back to the hospital. Perhaps she wants to prove to us that she really needs to go back. As I write this journal she keeps racing into my room, landing on the bed, talking for a few seconds, and then taking off again.

August 26

This place has a different character on weekends. During the week we can try to maintain the illusion that we are all part of the normal workaday world as we go to outpatient details, part-time jobs, school, and the like, but on weekends the illusion vanishes; we wait for phone calls, for word that we can go home for the day, for the weekend, for the week. The use of the phrase "go home" suggests that for many residents B Home is not really home, but rather a place to go (or to be sent) to when one can't live at home. Jerry put it simply: "I'm here because my parents don't want me at home anymore."

Jerry called me sweetheart and planted another kiss on my cheek. Rosa gasped, obviously shocked, but Jerry said it was just a kiss for luck. His statement defined things nicely. Then Jerry asked me if I wanted to meet my future husband. He pointed to David Kent who was sitting nearby. Jerry's assumption was not so strange, since David and I had recently spent some time talking together. Other people, including Karl and Rosa, made small efforts to push us together. David, however, has effectively countered the matchmaking by retreating, avoiding, denying. What is surprising, though, is the fact that before we had exchanged a single word at B Home Jerry had hypothesized a relationship between us. There is something uncanny about that.

I have been having stomach pains since last night, and they've begun to color all my reactions. Nothing seems to help — eating or not eating, tea, Coke, lying down or sitting up. It is very depressing to be sick in this place. I'm sure I'll live, but I wonder whom I could go to if I weren't sure.

August 29

I rushed back again this afternoon in order to go to the Rustic Canyon Recreation Center. And again we didn't go. No explanation.

It would seem that regularly scheduled events are not regularly scheduled.

Karl talked to me for a little while before dinner. I wish I could pin down why talking to him always makes me feel so good. From what I can see he also has that effect on many other people living here. One explanation is that he never comes on with that "and how *are you?*" line. Rather, his remarks are about interesting things that have nothing to do with our being patients. He isn't condescending. When he throws his arms around someone who is feeling bad, it is a brotherly action rather than that of a doctor relating to a patient. Although he makes me feel special as a woman, he doesn't convey the seductive undertones I sense from Don.

September 2

Jerry invited Rosa and me to see his new apartment at the B Home Annex. He is proud of his new quarters. It is something of a privilege to be allowed to live there. The apartment is well furnished and includes a genuine living room for the two occupants. It requires slightly more independent functioning by its residents because it is separated from the main B Home complex.

On the way back we stopped at the local thrift shop. The volunteer was especially nice to Jerry, whom she seemed to know from an earlier meeting. Apparently, for a few patients like Jerry, there is some interaction on the local community level.

I think that our departure from B Home is forcing some people here for the first time to confront the real possibility of leaving. In general, that is not a bad thing, especially for someone like Rosa. But for Jerry, an alternative living arrangement doesn't seem feasible now. I wonder . . .

After dinner I went into the TV room. Tim asked, "Will you marry me?" When I said no, he responded characteristically, "Then will you go to the doughnut shop and have coffee with me?" At first I started to say no but then Larry volunteered to come along and we all went over. While we were there quite a few residents dropped in. It seems to be a favorite hangout, probably because the young people who work in the shop aren't put off by the occasional strange behavior or appearance of the residents. One of the young men employed there offered Jerry coffee in return for dancing to the music on the radio. Jerry was obviously pleased and flattered by the arrangement. He dances well.

At some point Leon said that he was happy for me that I was leaving, but also sad for the others. It struck me that his way of putting it was especially nice. Up until now the remarks made to me had induced a sense of guilt at leaving others behind, making it even more difficult for me to go.

September 3

Had a relapse of my intestinal trouble this morning. I am no longer sure it's a virus. Perhaps it's the food, or maybe a mismanaged response to leaving.

I am feeling genuinely depressed about going. It's hard to make other people realize that this feeling is totally unrelated to my equally intense happiness at going home again. A few people here have become my friends. I'll miss them, though in reality they are friends of Helen Summers, not of Helen Sonier. One of the most important personal (and professional) realizations I have made here has been that, although I feel that I have been quite close to several of my patients in the past, no therapist would ever be allowed the kind of intimacy I have experienced here. That thought makes me sad for the future. But while I've always known it on some level, I suppose there is value in my becoming aware of it so dramatically.

With these thoughts drifting through my mind I found myself wandering aimlessly for most of the day, much as in earlier days. I feel as if an invisible curtain has been partly drawn, and I suppose others are aware of it, too. People still greet me as usual but, with the exception of Paul, they do not intrude.

Karl mentioned my leaving several times in the last couple of days, expressing sadness at my forthcoming departure. But he doesn't make it burdensome for me; he tries to be optimistic about my future. He surely is different from Leon, whose major response to my leaving has been to find out how soon he could move someone into my bed. That made me feel unimportant. Don said all the right things, but he seemed impersonal because what he said sounded to me like a prerecorded message.

Bingo as usual, although indoors because of rain. I have come to depend on regular activities like that, especially on a long weekend. Long holidays here are regarded oppositely from the way they are viewed on the outside. Instead of one more day of fun, a holiday is merely an extension of an already long, depressing weekend.

I had a preview of the letdown of leaving when David Kent went. He left at an awkward time, with Karl alone and busy with dinner, but still he looked forlorn as he walked out, suitcase in hand. There should be some kind of community ritual to celebrate departure. It would be important not only for the person leaving, who seems to be suddenly dropped by the staff, but for the community as a whole. The people who know me best may know where I am going, but to others who may know me only by sight I have simply disappeared, perhaps to the hospital, perhaps just to the outside. Who knows? So far as those left behind know, the discharged resident may simply have died. I've felt uneasy about the fate of people who were on the missing list after leaving.

I had promised Herb a farewell game of pool. There was something different about the level of our relationship. It was as if my leaving prompted Herb to disclose more of himself to me. He spoke about his family, his children, where they lived, and what they did. Perhaps he was trying to create a firmer bond between us before it was too late. My style, in contrast, has been to withdraw somewhat before termination.

While we were playing I mentioned my plan to come back for a visit. Herb reacted by noting that everyone intends to come back but no one ever does. That's not entirely true, but I realized that what he was saying was probably more often true than not. He prepares himself for my departure with the expectation that this is our final exchange.

Later that day I left.

DEBRIEFING WITH B HOME STAFF

September 12

Dr. Farberow and Dr. Crockett entered and were introduced to those present: Mack and Gwen B., the owners, Don, Mary, and Karl. NLF explained the use of the tape recorder: ". . . it's mostly for us so that we will remember the things that are going to be discussed today. This meeting is for a purpose. We at the VA and at the SPC have been interested for a very long time in suicide." (He then explained the background of the Central Research Unit at the VA and the Suicide Prevention Center.)

NLF: You may recall a meeting at VA in which this type of study was described to you. You gave us signed permission to place in one of your homes, at some time or other in the next six months, a researcher who would spend a month or so with you. Now we have done that, and I wonder if one of you remembers signing this particular paper.

Don: Yes, it was at one of the sponsors' meetings.

NLF: Sometime within the past month a researcher did enter into your home, and he or she may still be here or may have left. I wonder if you can make a guess. There are a number of things we want to know. One of them is the kind of indication that the person was not who he said he was.

Don guessed David Kent. "He appeared to be a very well-mannered young man. Also it was the way he would talk to me; he talked to me a couple of times."

Don: Plus he did a lot of good.

Mary: Yes, he did, much more so than any other resident that we've had. He'd participate in everything that was going on here.

There was some discussion about whether or not Kent was on medication, but they decided that he was.

Don felt that it might be DS, another resident, because he functioned at a very high level.

Don: I thought he was a pretty "together" person, though it seems that he was diagnosed as having suicidal tendencies.

(Apparently, in guessing who he was, staff members respond to the one-month time limit, the suspected suicidal diagnosis, the patient's originating from Dr. Crockett's building, and the probability that the researcher was alert and helpful.)

Don also found it difficult to get auxiliary information (a "green sheet") from the hospital on DS and David Kent, and that kind of reticence made them suspect.

Don continued to stress his suspicion that the researcher was DS.

NLF explained that the study is not trying to find fault with any facility or person but is focused on learning about the experiences of a resident after discharge from a hospital.

Mack, the owner of B Home, emphasized that one other patient was found to be suicidal but "never in a million years" would they have suspected it. The day before he overdosed he had "paid his rent in cash."

NLF explained that a second researcher had been introduced into the home to record a second point of view. Karl suggested Miss Summers. Mary agreed that it might be Helen — she was going to college.

Mack suggested someone else, C. Others disagreed.

Don then returned to the guess of Helen Summers. She was there only a short while. She worked.

NLF: Why might it have been Helen Summers?

Mary: She was another person who was just "together."

Don: She stayed only a short time. She decided to go back to the dorm.

Mary: She was going back to school.

Don: She also helped people here. She was teaching some of the guys to read and write while she was here. And she more or less took the initiative. You can see an outstanding person like that.

Karl felt that the two researchers were among Kent, Summers, and DS. There was consensus on that point.

At this point Helen, David, and their social workers, Keith Froehlich and Sharon Gallagher, were summoned into the room. Greeting and introductions followed. There was agreement that the staff didn't suspect the researchers while they were at B Home. DKR made his presentation.

Helen brought up some positive experiences: the staff's including her in conversations, their waiting to hear her response to questions about how she was and summoning her to the office at her convenience, a staff member's meeting someone halfway, and choices at meals. Quality of meals is obviously a sensitive and prideful area for the owners. The style of serving, the punctuality, the choices, and the quality are well planned.

The next two topics discussed brought defensive responses from the staff. Mary responded to a plea to trust residents with a reminder of the responsibility she carries as a staff member; DKR insisted that if a resident has correctly performed a staff member's task, such as counting those boarding a bus, the correctness of his act should be acknowledged. Don responded to a comment on the swimming pool that there are number of reasons why residents don't join him in the pool. DKR's point was not that residents have to join, but rather that they should be invited.

Helen reported that seemingly small things matter seriously to residents.

Keith emphasized that the learning experience of the staff in the psychiatric ward where last summer's research was conducted was valuable, especially the emphasis on previously unnoticed details that could be improved.

The comments on lack of weekend activities stimulated discussion among staff and owners about what actually was happening on weekends that is, what activities were planned. The request for alternative activities should a scheduled activity be canceled brought the response that some residents wouldn't participate in an alternative activity. DKR's answer, again, was that we can't force people to participate in an activity (as in the pool) but that simply the effort of invitation (the open alternative) is appreciated by the residents. DKR repeated the point that some small events loom large in residents' eyes.

David: Mary, if you care about people, you're going to realize that those small things are the things that really count because they are the only things that make up the residents' lives. And you're going to care about the things that happen in their lives. You keep saying "small" or "these small things" and I don't think they are. I think you wouldn't be here if you thought they were small.

Mack said he went to the VA hospital to visit two or three former residents over a one-year period because he realized (as did their doctor) that his visits were important to them.

An extended discussion about medications followed. DKR noted that he had accumulated 20 Elavil tablets in his shaving kit. Mary responded that she could imagine the upset at B Home if his hoard had been discovered; she predicted that he would probably have gone back to the hospital. The handing out of pills to those who are on self-medication is designed to prevent residents from exchanging medications with one another, stealing, and forgetting to take them.

The purposes of weekly inspection are upkeep of the building and detection of flagrant abuses, such as leaving clothes lying around. Inspectors also have found pills on the dining room floor. Some residents are watched more closely than others, depending on their histories and their medication (e.g., Antabuse). If they neglect medication residents usually start slipping fast and become noticeable.

Mary said that, in retrospect. DKR's story wasn't very plausible.

Helen felt that the kind of attention she needed from others varied during the course of her stay at B Home. Too much heartiness, coming on strong, caused her to withdraw. Being perceptive to the proper pacing was helpful.

DKR: How did you see us?

Mary: I don't think we had much trouble picking you out because you were so "together." You participated and you helped.

Karl had suspected that perhaps both DKR and HS were on LSD. He knew by appearance that neither of them was mentally disturbed. Karl thought their way of walking, with swinging arms and open faces, was too normal.

Mary said she had thought that Kent didn't belong at B Home. She had checked his history and had discovered he was suicidal, and she had been suspicious of his story (but she said that often she gets distorted stories from residents so she didn't think much about it). She had planned to check further.

Mack emphasized that he spends perhaps an extra $20,000 in ten years to ensure good-quality food — "It's little." He also talked about the new facility bus and new carpeting for all apartments. He realized that putting new carpeting in some apartments and not in others would create bad feelings.

Helen pointed out that there is a system of mutual assistance among residents. Mary agreed that they help on a low level and participate sometimes, but not so consistently as Kent and Summers did.

Mack wasn't sure what day Helen had left, but he knew she had paid until September 4. He also pointed out that for about the last week of David's and Helen's stay one staff member was on vacation, and so the management was shorthanded.

DKR asked about staff members who spend considerable time with residents of the opposite sex. Don felt that females are usually the ones who want to talk a lot. Mary felt it was natural to deal with more men because "we have so many more men than women."

Don: We deal with people as they come, male or female.

NLF suggested that the practice is based mainly on need, and the staff agreed.

NLF: What do you see as the primary objectives and goals of the board-and-care home? What are you aiming for? What are your purposes?

Gwen: To give them a home and to make them comfortable as long as they need us. That's my aim.

Don saw the home as a "stepping-stone to the community," or, in other words, as supportive care. "After the hospital brings patients to a certain level, we should give them the added boost they need to put them back into the community. Of course, we're going to provide homes for some people, too. You wouldn't eliminate the fact that there are some people who simply need homes. For them, this place will be about the closest to the community they're going to get."

There was some feeling that new state laws were being used as an excuse to empty psychiatric facilities into board-and-care facilities. As a result the residents (even VA ex-patients) are sicker than before.

Don: Well, we really wouldn't want the home to be a hospital, and we don't want to be a place that's just warehousing people. We would like to keep on making progress. But if we get a person who is not at the necessary level, either he has to go back into the hospital or we have to keep him and deal with him here. And so conditions might necessitate a long-term stay here, and that might appear to be warehousing, but it's not.

Don wasn't in favor of sending a person back to the hospital unless necessary, but he felt strongly that such persons ought not to be released from the hospital in the first place. Prevention is fine. But if some of the residents were better "leveled-off" with medication they would be easier to deal with in the board-and-care home.

Putting a resident back into the VA hospital seems to be a problem area. Sometimes the person is again released almost immediately. The jurisdiction of the wards may be clearly spelled out on paper, but the practice of getting an ex-patient readmitted presents difficulties, particularly with the night shift.

Don: A lot of times there's controversy in the ward. So you're bickering back and forth about where a certain patient should go. And he's standing there listening to you. . . . It just makes you want to scream. Makes you wonder who is really sick.

Dr. Crockett mentioned an example of Don's cooperation with the hospital in rescuing a suicidal resident at B Home while her psychologist kept her talking on another line.

Don: We try to gear our activities to the home community. For example, we had to discontinue a barbershop we had here because the guys stopped going to the barbershop outside. We've tried different things and discontinued them for a good reason.

Mack asked the researchers their opinion of the canteen. They had found it useful. It functioned differently from coffee shops on the outside. Helen pointed out that it was run by the patients for their own profit. It was a good get-together place. Mack reported that he had spent $2,000 to set up the canteen. He pays for electricity for its daily operation.

We inquired about the reasonableness of telling the residents about our study. The response was positive: "It might give them a boost." Probably a few would feel spied upon. The staff worried that it might compromise our next project if we encountered some of these same residents elsewhere. "Do you think there might be fears of new residents coming in? That they might not be accepted?" "You can't protect them. They've got to face reality." Mary wanted to know if there was a positive reason for telling the residents about the researchers. The latter expressed concern that residents might find out anyway from an indirect source. The researchers also found it difficult to return to B Home for further contacts while maintaining the fiction of their cover. Finally, letting the residents in on the research and asking for their perspectives would be useful both for the study and for the residents. Because their opinions would be seen as worthwhile, telling them would help to build a positive self concept.

DKR and HS agreed to speak to the residents at dinner the following night. Mack invited the researchers to eat with the residents as the guests of B Home.

DEBRIEFING WITH B HOME RESIDENTS

September 13

The meeting was held in the dining room after many of the residents had begun to eat. Most of them stopped eating to listen when it was announced that someone was going to speak.

DKR presented an outline of the research project. This public presentation was aimed at countering the possibility that residents would hear about the experiment from other sources. Even those who couldn't hear clearly were aware that a public statement had been made. Some residents checked later with other residents, staff members, and the researchers about the details.

The emphasis in the announcement was on the researchers' living the residents' life, the genuineness of their friendships with the residents, and the potential benefit to them. It was announced that DKR and HS would be at poolside until 6 P.M. so that those who were interested could talk with them and see that basically they remained the same down-to-earth people the residents had known before. Don emphasized that the management had not known the alternate identities of David and Helen before yesterday.

At poolside a number of residents, usually in twos and threes, came over to shake hands and talk about the research and the recent news around the facility. One man wanted to protest that the rent is too high when four to six residents are crowded into one apartment. He also said that the light in his ceiling had been fixed after he had complained, but that the lights in several other apartments were not working. When he asked for pictures for the walls of his room he got them, but others didn't have any.

The reactions of all who met with the two former residents were positive and interested. Arrangements were made to meet people later to study together, play chess, and talk.

COMPARISON OF EXPERIENCES

Placement of two researchers as participant-observers in the same environment at the same time enabled us to observe similarities and differences in the two experiences. Did the researchers validate each other? Or were the experiences contrasting? Examination of the two journal accounts reveals many more similarities than differences.

Helen's residence in B Home was her first experience in such a role, and she was obviously much more anxious and ill than was Kent. It took her a number of days — in fact, almost a full week — before she could feel relaxed and less concerned that she was playing her role adequately, and before she could feel comfortable (less frightened) with the displays of delusional and hallucinatory behavior about her. Kent had had previous experience as a suicidal patient, within a setting where much stricter scrutiny prevailed. The stay in B Home placed no severe strain on him; all he had to do was avoid isolation and boredom, if possible. Indeed, boredom and inactivity (especially on weekends) were common aspects of existence for both Helen and David.

Another marked similarity appears in their reactions to being residents. The sense of second-class citizenship became very strong for both of them, just as it does for patients in the hospital. Staff-resident interactions took on a special significance; staff members assumed an adversary role resembling parental authority. Both researchers had had expectations of being taken care of, of being directed, of being organized and guided by the staff, and so they found themselves becoming angry at the detachment characterizing some of the staff. Alliances were formed with other residents instead of with staff. And these alliances often served as crucial sources of information and of emotional support. Each researcher reacted positively to behavior signaling humanistic respect, as in interactions with Karl, and negatively to disregard or lack of consideration, as when Rustic Canyon trips were canceled without notification.

Another strong feeling Helen and David shared about being residents was the realization of powerlessness, impressed upon them both directly and subtly. The mechanical pronouncements of interest from the staff, the asking of questions without bothering to wait for answers, the delays or absences of response to the expressed needs of residents — all were very irritating. The researchers also recognized the expectation of the staff that residents would stay in the facility and not move on into the community as a subtle confirmation of their need for continuous help and for a protective environment.

Helen had far more difficulty than Kent in learning the routine. No information was available as to the schedule for activities and meals; one had to seek out the information for oneself or else miss out on many things. Kent actively explored the situation, whereas Helen learned rather slowly and tentatively in the midst of her tension and anxiety.

Both Helen and Kent reported on the meals in full detail. Obviously the lack of entertaining activities heightened the importance of the three regular events of the day: breakfast, lunch, and dinner. Food had more significance for Kent than for Helen. He found himself living the role of resident so fully that he became almost childish about the mechanics of eating: he rushed to get to the dining room early; he disliked losing his place at the table and "sharing" his food; he gulped down his meals just as fast as the others did. Helen, however, at first showed little interest in the food; she enjoyed the relationships with others at her table and would have liked to linger with a cigarette over her coffee, but she couldn't because smoking was prohibited in the dining room.

Concern with selfhood was strong in both researchers. NOVA was important to Kent. He appreciated the effort to help residents become more involved in determining their status and function.

NOVA gave the residents a chance to meet, share their concerns, and develop a unified program for modification of factors affecting their lives. Helen never mentioned NOVA, and we assume she did not attend any of the meetings. She crocheted, and reacted with real anger when a staff member was inappropriately effusive over her work. The comment, which seemed condescending to her, gave her the impression that she was a child being patted on the head. Helen's anger centered on the staff attitude that former mental patients were just not expected to be creative and competent.

Both researchers noted that certain kinds of interactions with staff members prompted impulses toward acting "crazy." Cues that they were expected to remain permanent residents in the setting prompted feelings of despair and aroused the urge to indulge in inappropriate acting out. Similarly, when other residents were perceived to be incorrectly viewing the researchers' normal behavior as abnormal, the indignation sparked fantasies of retaliatory craziness. Finally, being ignored and treated as nonpersons evoked impulses toward various forms of attention-seeking behavior. Of course, we are not the first to document the fact that others' behavior can elicit abnormal behavior from those labeled insane. Braginsky et al. (1969), Goffman (1961), and Laing (1961), for example, have reported similar findings.

Stages in the resident's career. — Both Helen and Kent passed through a sequence of loosely defined stages during their residency in B Home. The stages are described in detail in Reynolds and Farberow (1976).

The first stage in the resident's career is the "newcomer status." Helen and David were new faces. They were greeted, introduced, noticed, welcomed. They quickly learned that the question "Where are you from?" usually did not mean "What state were you born in?" or "What part of the country did you live in?" but "What hospital were you discharged from?" The name of the hospital and, more specifically, the ward to which one had been assigned are important factors in determining social links or a basis of shared experience with others.

As in most settings, certain privileges were accorded the newcomers. They were allowed to be ignorant of rules. They were permitted to ask many questions, sometimes repetitiously. Criticism for inappropriate behavior was temporarily suspended while the new residents made their adjustment to the new life.

The next phase the researchers passed through is the "interim phase." Newcomer status wears off in time and the resident enters the interim phase, regarded as one of the most dangerous stages for the potentially suicidal patient. Kent's novelty value declined over time. He began to note with jealousy the greetings expressed to more recent newcomers. And he noticed the stereotypical quality of these greetings. He had not been someone special after all, but just another marionette in a long life of newcomers who enjoyed the spotlight and then suffered in the shadows.

> I had not made friends yet; I hadn't even learned the names of my peers. I had merely enjoyed passively the attention I got. Now I was in limbo. Contact with my friends in the psychiatric ward was cut off. New relationships in this aftercare facility were still hazy and unripe.
>
> Furthermore, I hadn't yet learned the niches, the lifeways, possible in a board-and-care home. And it looked as if I was going to be there a long time. No one had begun talking to me about my return to society as they had from my first day in the hospital. I was expected to stay. This place was no stepping-stone to the outside world. It was a warehouse for storing away society's rejects.
>
> No longer dazed by my new surroundings, I began to compare myself with the other residents. The apathy of my fellows disturbed me. I overheard a resident being asked how old he was. "Thirty-seven," he responded. It struck me that in six years I, too, would be like him. All around me I saw walking previews of things to come in my life.
>
> Comparisons with those who appeared to be in better shape than I was also produced despondency. Those who seemed to interact confidently and smoothly with the female residents especially underscored my own shyness and hesitancy in this area. In the psychiatric ward from which I came there has been no women, though of course there were female nurses and nursing assistants. But they were so closely bound to their roles that I never saw them as socially acceptable companions. Suddenly I found myself in a small, confined society with women, some young and pretty. But though they were nearby spatially, they were unreachable.
>
> In my journal I wrote: "As I withdraw a bit this morning, lying in bed, the sounds of activity outside my room mock me and emphasize the difference between me and the others. How can they care so little, to be able to go on with their lives while I am sad, not even wondering why I'm not among them? Such is the self-centeredness of the depressed." (Reynolds, 1975)

Nevertheless, Helen and David moved through this interim period and progressed to the stage of real membership in the aftercare community. They began to know individuals, to have expectations, and to gain a sense of what was just and what was unjust within the accepted norms of the facility. An example will illustrate the experience of being drawn into the web of interrelationships among the residents. At breakfast one morning Kent tried to switch cereals, but when the resident who arrived shortly afterward claimed his own cereal back, Kent reluctantly gave it to him. To get even, Kent passed the milk pitcher away from the resident to the other end of the table. His opponent had to ask Kent to pass the milk. This kind of trivial childishness was a signal that Kent was being drawn into social relationships of sufficient depth to pull affective reactions from him.

The resident who has adapted to life in a board-and-care facility has a number of options or niches into which he can fit himself. For example, there is the gamester who is expert at all sorts of games, from chess and checkers to bridge, pinochle, tennis, Ping-Pong, and pool. His day is spent playing or organizing games. Another resident hangs out at a local doughnut shop where his informal relations with the help occasionally enable him to exchange light cleanup work or entertainment for free coffee and doughnuts. Other residents are hustlers who arrange dinner dates and other activities with the women residents. Escapists of several kinds utilize television, sleep, reading, hallucinations, alcohol, movies, and even church activities to keep them psychologically, if not physically, away from the facility for much of the day.

Looking back on their stay in the facility, both researchers could see why it was an ending point, a cul-de-sac, for many residents. The rewards of life were simple but reasonable and the demands were very few. It was a sheltered world of acquaintance-peers with whom they did not need to compete. There was a benevolent authority to whom they could appeal in the event of trouble — and then hope for action. Within very broad limits (including financial and medical limits) their freedom of movement was unrestricted. There were irritations, to be sure: disturbances caused by fellow residents, the occasional insensitivity of management, the limitations on personal space, and an erratic schedule of activities. But these were relatively minor if the resident was able to lower his aspirations and trim his potential to fit the rewards offered by the system. It was not a bad place to live, it was only a terribly limiting one. Thus it is not surprising that few residents actually reach the point of terminating residency in such a facility.

Those who do decide to leave the facility can be expected to have doubts about their ability to make it on the outside. A kind of temporary prestige accrues to the resident who is about to move out on his own. Yet his peers begin to disengage, too, as they realize that he isn't likely to return again — unless he fails. His thoughts begin to turn toward his new life in the larger community. The prospective change fills his conversations; even before he goes, the social world of those he is leaving behind begins to mend the hole he will make in the social fabric by leaving. On the day that Kent actually left he felt a sharp sense of anticlimax. Few people seemed to acknowledge or even notice his going. The one bright spot was his recollection that earlier in the week two staff members had given him their home phone numbers should he have trouble and need to talk with someone. And there was a clear understanding that he would be welcome should he decide to return, and perhaps even an expectation that he would return.

During her last days in the facility, Helen found herself just wandering about, withdrawn into her thoughts of leaving and receiving a variety of messages from those around her. Staff responded with businesslike plans, prerecorded therapy messages, and genuine concern. Residents backed away or opened up in a final effort to achieve intimacy.

Both researchers felt the need for a communal ceremony at leaving, for recognition of the event and the progress it represented. Such a ceremony would be token community support and good wishes.

Another route for leaving the board-and-care home is the one that leads back to the hospital. Several residents during Helen's and Kent's stay asked to go back to the protected haven of their former psychiatric wards. Several others wanted so badly to go back that they caused trouble, thus inviting rehospitalization.

The career cycle may be renewed when a resident who left on his own comes back. The cutback in welfare payments when one leaves a board-and-care home presents the newly independent ex-resident with an immediate problem. Understandably, some persons see the reduction in funds as punishment for leaving. The scarcity of money, compounded by the lack of skills related to living alone — skills such as cooking, budgeting time, finding and holding a job, handling money, dealing with physical illness — may make life on the outside more trouble than it is worth. Of equal importance is the unbearable loneliness on the outside. As one resident who came back to the home said, "You start talking to strangers in the park and they have other people to talk to and other things to talk about."

Neither Helen nor Kent experienced an immediate return to the hospital environment (although Kent subsequently lived in several other aftercare residences), but they observed and interacted with others representing each of the stages described above. There was much to learn from their peers, for the residents themselves are the experts in this lifeway.

The conceptual importance of the successive stages — newcomer, interim, membership, termination — is discussed in the final section of this book, where suggestions and recommendations are made. In brief, we believe that preparing the resident for these phases helps reduce the perplexity of passing through them. Here we wish to emphasize the recognition of the two researchers that such a career pathway exists in B Home. Subsequent investigation revealed its existence in all the residential aftercare facilities with which we are familiar.

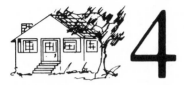4

L HOME

The second aftercare facility we studied, L Home, is much smaller than B Home. It has the capacity to house fifteen residents, both men and women. At the time, however, only men were living there. A social worker described the facility as follows: "A large older building in good repair. Near shopping area, schools, churches, etc. The VA Outpatient Clinic is nearby. The sponsor is a friendly and cooperative person who has great interest and concern for the people in her care. She is a middle-aged RN and has worked at various health-related jobs for many years. She also has had a number of years' experience in operating a board-and-care home. Nearly any type of patient may be placed in this facility." Another social worker called L Home "one of the best homes available."

KENT'S L HOME JOURNAL

November 17

I arrived at L Home a bit after 2 P.M. My social worker, Keith, brought me here, along with my suitcase and sack. I had about $14 spending money in addition to my first month's rent.

Today it was difficult to induce depression. My usual tactics — fixed downward gaze, slumping shoulders, repetitions of my story with emphasis on the hopelessness of my future, sighs, shallow breathing, even sitting for half an hour in the ward — were relatively ineffective. Since my mood rhythm cycle was high, the best I could do was exhibit slowness and quietness and build on the anxiety and fear associated with the newness and the unknown elements of today. By the time we arrived I was nervous, anxious, cautious, and passively willing to agree to anything.

The neighborhood is lower middle class, near the Los Angeles civic center. The home is a large, white, two-story boardinghouse, old but clean and well kept up. The homelike setting is clearly established with a comfortably furnished living room, a TV room, a dining room, and bedrooms and bathrooms upstairs. There are individual rooms but also "family" rooms. We went into the living room where Keith introduced me to Mrs. B. I may have been told earlier that Mrs. B. is black, but when I was introduced to her my first reaction was to see the complications of living and researching here. In the first few moments it was clear that Mrs. B.'s role as a mothering person dominates other roles; she is a very nice lady. I also met Allen, her seven-year-old son, in the first few minutes. The boy (and perhaps also his sister) is an important socializer in this setting. First, his presence communicates trust. He needs care from adults, and his dependency (I tied his cap strings at Mrs. B.'s request) is natural and nonemasculating, to him or to us, because he's a child.

I was shown to my room upstairs. It is furnished with a bed, chair, and dresser for each of the two occupants. There are pictures, a decorated plate, and a mirror on the walls and a rug on the floor.

Mrs. B. gave me three towels, a washcloth, two bars of soap, and a box of tissues. She said that my roommate had left the home and wondered if it bothered me to sleep alone in a room. I replied that I didn't care. Then she turned to Keith and asked what he thought about bringing in a roommate to be with me. "It's up to you," she said to him. They would decide for me, but only after asking me. I passively assented to anything. After a few minutes Keith left with Mrs. B.

I put away my things and lay down on the bed. In about ten or fifteen minutes Mrs. B. knocked on my door and came in. She asked a few questions about my past. After learning that I liked to watch TV, she promised to bring me a television set on Monday. She said that she was of a different race but that among friends color doesn't matter. And she wanted to be my friend.

She asked if I was a Catholic. This question, like several others she asked, was aimed at establishing a sense of mutuality between us. She explained that she, too, had lost her parents and also a husband and a son in the war and another husband by separation. Allen's birthday was about a week away from mine. The purpose of the conversation seemed to be to establish commonalities. In response to her query about my faith, I said that I wasn't "anything." She said that I just meant I didn't adhere to any religion. She feels I'm "something," that I'm young and have to learn to accept losses and keep my head up.

She wants me to think of this place as my home, but she'll be working to get me into my own apartment quickly. "You've got a friend," she said. More important, she showed me that I did indeed have a friend by promising a TV on Monday, bringing a radio on Saturday, buying me coffee and pie on our trip that afternoon, planning to get me a jacket as part of my Christmas present, and letting me know that if I'm low in money or can't pay rent, I can stay anyway. (One resident hasn't paid for two years. Mrs. B. obviously isn't profit-oriented, at least in an economic sense.)

She asked if I'd go with her and Allen to get his eyes checked. While waiting in the living room I was introduced to Rick, a resident. He said that L Home is the best, or one of the best, family-care facilities. Without being pushy, he offered information about the location of stores and a park. Also, I found myself involved in plans to go to the racetrack with Rick and Mrs. B. Later that day plans were also made for future trips for shopping and movies. I wasn't left alone to get lonely and work up a depression. Already I was caught up in natural positive relationships with others in this setting.

Another social worker came by and offered us a lift to the doctor's office. While waiting, Mrs. B. treated me to coffee and pie in a nearby coffee shop. Obviously well known in the area, she was greeted cordially by the elevator operator, the doctor's receptionist, a short-order cook, the coffee shop manager, and a couple of people we passed in the street. She has lived in this area seven or eight years.

Mrs. B. began early to establish herself in my eyes as competent and caring. She cited her experiences in raising many children and caring for many veterans. Several former residents now have apartments in the neighborhood. She visits them to see that they are continuing their medication. She felt certain she could help me. "You'll see," she said with confidence. She calls some residents "baby" and speaks of her "boys" and her "children" when referring to them. And even with strangers she calls this her "home." When I became cold walking outside in the chilling wind, she tried to find us a cab and even put her shawl around my shoulders.

She believes that her home can be a stepping-stone for young people like me. But I can stay as long as necessary. At this point she could have said almost anything about my problem and my future and I would have been inclined to go along with it. She is a really beautiful person, naturally saying and doing much of what is precisely "right."

After the doctor's examination we went downstairs to pick out Allen's glasses. We passed a young girl with one leg. "You need only look around you to see how well off you are," commented Mrs. B. She and Allen asked for my opinion when selecting the frame for the glasses.

We walked to a hamburger stand (no taxi in sight) where she ordered fifteen hamburgers and bags of potato chips and two pies. Buying prepared food is no way to guarantee profits in residential care, but the appointment with the eye doctor had cut into her cooking time. The pace was a bit brisk. This neighborhood is an interesting one with lots going on. It has movies, parks, businesses, stores of all kinds, and a fascinating melange of inner-city people. Mrs. B's expectations of me were a bit high. I had trouble walking so fast and talking simultaneously. Furthermore, she seemed to think I would be familiar with directions and routes after she pointed them out and we walked them just once. Most of the time I kept my eyes on the ground.

On our return I went up to my room and soon was called to dinner. We are called to each meal personally (sometimes twice by a considerate neighbor). The meals are served family style at three small tables. There is chatter at the tables, and the atmosphere is relaxed and is marked by an attitude of sharing. Mrs. B. asked us when we wanted to eat supper regularly and explained why this one, at 5:50 P.M., was so late. I was introduced to all the residents and heard for the second time that George wasn't at supper because he had a chest cold and was resting in his room. Mrs. B. joked about having to kick some guys to keep them up and active, but she works with love and frankness rather than punishment, and everyone here knows it. I also met her daughter who seems to be about eleven years old.

After dinner I took a bath in the old, but clean, tub and got into bed. Shortly afterward Mrs. B. knocked on the door. We talked for a while. She asked if I was living alone when I made my suicide attempt, adding that it's not good to be alone. If I want a haircut (she knows I wouldn't want her barber to do it), she'll give me money to pay for it. She promised to call me later that night if I wanted her to, but I said I was going right to sleep.

She explained that she inspects our rooms once a week because of health regulations; that there's a fire drill occasionally, even at 2 A.M., a time when there might be a fire; that each resident is required to take a daily bath; that naps should be short if taken at all; and that it helps if we make our beds but we don't have to. Again she emphasized that because I'm good looking, intelligent, and young I shouldn't lie around but ought to get out. "Of course, as long as you're here it's money in my pocket," she laughed. She gave me a receipt for my rent.

Mrs. B. said her son would be disappointed that I wasn't going home with them that night. They live a few miles away. He told her that I could be his doctor (?). There's a night watchman here, and she'd see that I got her phone number. She warned me that one resident might pace at night, and also that she sometimes needs to shout at people but that I shouldn't get upset by such events. "See you in the morning," and she left.

I slept from 7:30 until 7 A.M. My dreams had three memorable features. First, I dreamed of being taken care of and of being fed. Second, I dreamed of being schizophrenic with hallucinations and amnesia; I nearly cried when I realized it. Third, I dreamed that a nurse knew her patient's habits so well that she knew when he would vomit and provided him with an emesis pan shortly before he needed it.

I learned later from Mrs. B. that she came to the home at 2 A.M. and prayed by each person's door, a not infrequent event.

November 18

I got up and washed. I saw Mrs. B. scrubbing in the bathroom. I was called to breakfast about 8:30. At the breakfast table Mrs. B. said she had noticed on my referral form that I was a writer. She said I ought to write about "Mrs. B.'s family," but I ought to visit other places, too, so I'd have some perspective. She said that she's been here a long time and has never had serious problems and never has heard a complaint about food. She has no strict rules, feeling that adults don't need them. (The daily bath requirement seems like a rule to me.) Everyone gets along well together. She allows beer or wine if it is drunk in moderation. And we're welcome to bring friends here.

Sometimes she yells, she warns me; she has to kick tails now and then but it keeps her shoes shined.

She spoke of her trip to Hawaii with several of the residents. They took medications along, but no one needed pills because there was so much to do. At the table one fellow quipped that he'd have to go to the kitchen to get a second cup of coffee because the coffee wasn't strong enough to come out to him.

After breakfast Mrs. B. came up to my room and had me fill out a simple background data sheet. Again, she searched for commonalities. I don't eat much, neither does she; we both like to bathe before going to bed, and so on.

She invited me to go shopping, but I said that I wanted to watch football on TV. She had work to do and went off. I sat reading. Later I was called to the telephone. Mrs. B. had wanted to say good-bye before she left but didn't have the chance. "Have you been asleep?" she asked. "No," I replied. "Do you want to go to a movie?" she asked. "No."

A black resident stood in the hallway talking to himself: "Make him grow, Hollywood. Teach him all about California. Know how to change a diaper? Put his li'l white gown on him." I imagined he'd lost his wife and baby.

I watched football alone all afternoon. Mrs. B. came in for a few minutes. She brought me a book about depression and suggested we might discuss it later. She has a "suicidal" over at the other place, but she thinks I'm not one. She has faith that I won't take too many pills, but she exacted my promise that I wouldn't. She asked if I wanted to go with her, but I preferred to watch TV. She inquired about my food preferences, noting I hadn't eaten much for lunch. She also remarked that 25 milligrams of Elavil twice a day isn't a heavy dose, so the doctor must think I don't need much. "The others will warm up to you in time," she assured me.

I wrote notes from 3:30 to 4:30 P.M. Then came supper. The cook asked me, "Is that all you can put away, Hon?" but she seemed satisfied with my effort to eat. I had remarked at breakfast that I preferred milk to coffee, and thereafter there was always a glass of milk at my place. After supper I went back to watch TV until 9:30 P.M. Alone, I began to feel neglected. Strange, before I felt smothered and now I felt abandoned. I bathed and got ready for bed. Wrote notes until 10:45 P.M.

November 19

Up at 6:45 A.M., washed my face, and made the bed. I listened to the radio which Mrs. B. brought me yesterday. Mrs. B. knocked on the door as I sat slumped in my chair in the darkened room.

I told her I hadn't slept well last night. She said that I was looking better, that I was holding my head up higher than yesterday. (I didn't believe it.) She said I was too young for sleeping pills, and she doesn't believe that pills can make a person sleep anyway. I'm welcome to heat up milk at night; there's no rule about staying out of the kitchen. "Guys who come here from board-and-care facilities sometimes think they have to stay in their rooms all day," she said, "but here we have a living room and radios downstairs. It's a real home." She knows I wouldn't use a knife to hurt myself. She doesn't trust people (she trusts only God), but she has faith in them. Sometimes people disappoint us, sometimes we disappoint ourselves, but we always hope for the best. She asked if I had an electric razor. I told her I wanted to grow a beard because my face is becoming irritated from shaving. She thought I'd look like those young doctors at USC with long hair and beards we were talking about at lunch yesterday.

Mrs. B. offered to do my laundry for me. She asked if I was beginning to feel better. She wanted me to be in charge of answering the phone downstairs tomorrow. And Tuesday we'd go to her other place for a visit. She wanted to know if she was pushing me too fast and if I felt lonely. I said I was used to being alone. Having taken my wastebasket to empty, she left. During our talk I was upset; I shed a few tears, swallowed back a lump in my throat, sighed, and kept my eyes averted. Mrs. B.'s interest and hopefulness didn't flag, however.

At the table Sarah insisted on giving me both milk and coffee when I hesitated over which to have. She asked how I wanted my eggs. Daryl, seated at my table, kindly passed the sugar and cream (remembering I take both), offered apple butter and pepper (after I'd reached for salt). People greeted and took care of me. As Mrs. B. said, "They know you're a man but here you're a baby, the youngest one." There was joking about several guys who were "shacking up" with women or who might go out on their own if Mrs. B. could find gals for them to live with. The consensus was that in California it's acceptable to live that way. The banter built a sense of masculinity.

There was talk of what movies are playing nearby. Rick wanted his dinner held if he returned late from a movie. That arrangement was fine. An astounding place! Really, it is more like a "home" than a "business." But what rare people are Mrs. B. and her cook!

After ten minutes in my room Larry called me. Mrs. B. wanted to talk with me outside. She was watering the lawn while we talked for about half an hour. The world was huge and the sun was bright after I had spent a full day shut up in the house. Just walking about inside the fenced yard made me feel as though I were on a trip. Mrs. B. talked about her lawn and her gardening, about improvements in the neighborhood initiated because she had started fixing her place up, and about the teenage parolees she used to keep here. She still keeps contact with those young people, some of whom have become teachers, some housewives; one is a postman, another a policeman. They come to visit her on Mother's Day and Christmas. She's proud of their achievements. Sometimes she stays up half the night reading and thinking about young people and their problems.

Mrs. B. showed simple politeness in thanking Larry for a small service he performed. She excused herself when going in to answer the phone and apologized when the hose accidentally pulled across my shoe. The social niceties demonstrate that in her eyes we are worthy social beings.

She talked about my getting my apartment with someone else. I told her that my friend might let me move in with him. She said he could visit here and even stay overnight anytime. She hoped I didn't mind the kidding around and noise at breakfast. Everyone likes me and they're just trying to get me to smile and be happy. People get along well here. Daryl, another resident, walks Mrs. B.'s children to school and brings them home every day. He wants to do it for them.

Mrs. B. is using the mild interest that Allen has in me, exaggerating it a bit and hoping to build a tie between the two of us. She told me that when Allen's new teacher at school asked him how many brothers and sisters he had, he replied, "Eighteen in one house and ten in another." Mrs. B.'s children think of us as family members. But I'm young and Allen thinks I'm a child, too. Living with all sorts of people has given her children quite an education. Mrs. B. attributes her daughter's A grades in a strict Catholic school in part to this living experience. She said Allen wanted to phone me (later he was on the phone but didn't want to talk to me, though she covered it up). She wanted to bring him by this afternoon to see me. "OK?" she asked. I nodded. She again pointed out the directions of several streets and the approximate location of the college I plan to attend. Such repetition is helpful.

I thanked her for talking with me and started upstairs, but she wanted to show me another son's photo. The boy was killed in the navy. She also spoke of the little girl who "expired." She knew how I felt, losing someone. She had needed others to help her through the crises or she might have ended up in a hospital, too.

She and Sarah love me. I'm young, and they are both mothers and know how to make me feel better. Her "boys" are pampered and spoiled but she'd rather have it that way.

Again I started back upstairs but she asked if I had read the Sunday paper yet. I came back and sat in the living room reading the *Herald-Examiner.* It contained pictures of a man jumping to his death.

Daryl left, looking good in a suit and tie. Mrs. B., Sarah, and Glen remarked on his appearance. They knew he'd decided, after all, to go to church. (He likes to put a dollar on the collection plate, but since he doesn't have the money today he was in doubt at breakfast whether or not to go.) "I wish you'd bring her back and let me see her," Mrs. B. kidded him. We all appreciated her quip, perhaps Daryl most of all.

Glen read the paper, too, made some appropriate comments, and then stood in the downstairs hallway talking aloud to no one. He was hallucinating. No one paid any attention to him.

Periodically, the television picture lost its focus, requiring me to get up to adjust it. I wonder how much exercise could be assured by manufacturing television sets and radios that require frequent adjustment, putting stairways in facilities, and finding naturally occurring simple tasks with which residents could help.

At lunchtime we had no lunch. I was worried that I'd been forgotten or that no one had called me, but later I learned, by overhearing Glen's soliloquy, that we get only two meals on Sunday.

I went upstairs and sat on the screened porch, reading and watching the "outside" for awhile. I watched a Mexican American woman walk down the street with a large bundle on her back. For many women life consists primarily in bearing things — packages, children, sorrow, the weight of a man.

Tomorrow I must handle the phone. I dread it. What ought I to do? What if I fail? It's a heavy responsibility to answer the phone for a whole day.

I went downstairs to watch TV. Doc, another resident, was already there so I watched the programs he selected. A commercial advertising candy bars stimulated me to go out to buy one. Doc gave directions. No one remarked on my leaving as I went out the front door. I selected the candy and paid the storekeeper without a word. He thanked me automatically. With my fledgling beard and my stigmatized status it felt good to be treated as just another customer. In this neighborhood, in contrast with a conservative middle-class community, I imagine the storekeeper sees all kinds of people and must accept them in order to stay in business.

November 20

The undermining of initiative and activity had begun. I was content to just sit. One tempting aspect of resident status is the opportunity to match activities to one's inner mood. In my other world, I (like most people in our society) have to subordinate my impulses and whims to the business of clock-oriented work and play. Here the time constraints and the behavior required of me are minimal. Perhaps a leisurely life style is more suited to man's biological nature. If so, it's no wonder that we have trouble pulling people away from environments like this one. And if doing little were culturally accept-able — as it well may be a hundred years from now — how different would our lives be from the lives of people here in this home? If we can go beyond the middle-class aversion to this life style, we begin to see that it holds advantages, such as a comfortable community life and a kind of freedom not enjoyed by many other role groups.

At breakfast Mrs. B. asked if she had given me a cup so I could conveniently take the prescribed pills in my room. She thought of it last night. "See, I'm thinking about you guys all the time." Daryl holds that Mrs. B. can see and hear what's going on here no matter where she is. Hmmmmmmmmm.

After breakfast I went into the living room, sat down by the telephone, and began to read. There was laughter and talk in the dining room. Mrs. B. came in and asked if I was warm enough. She bustled around, turned on a light so I could read better and, as always, communicated her concern both verbally and nonverbally. In the dining room she talked (for my benefit?) of the stiff licensing inspections she always passes. She told the cook that it's a good sign when residents feel free to complain because then you know what they like.

I started upstairs to brush my teeth. Mrs. B. noticed my leaving and speculated that her talk bothered me. "I'll have to keep my mouth shut." It wasn't so, but I was too tired to explain why I was leaving the room.

Allen came up to my room with his parochial school reader. "Where is God?" he asked. He paused for just a moment. "Every-where," he said, smiling, and left. Again I felt that Mrs. B. had sent him. (She said later that she hadn't.) He came up again to say good-bye: "Have a nice day." Again, he gave a big smile, turned quickly, and disappeared down the stairs.

I went back downstairs. As usual, soothing music undulated from the living room radio. I noticed that my lips were pursed — holding back, holding in — just as the rest of my body and my mind were turned in on myself. I realized that, since the phones are downstairs, keeping my eye on them requires the resident to come down from his room. Here is another example of naturally contrived situational pressures requiring (indirectly) some activity.

Mrs. B. is doing so much for me that I feel some pressure to reciprocate. The phone answering is fairly simple. It was mentioned yesterday, but no one applied pressure (or even brought it up) today. If I acted on the suggestion, it was going to be on my own initiative.

Daryl went out for a bottle. He brought one back last night, too. He'll be visiting his sister again soon, and Mrs. B. will give him extra money to buy good clothes before he goes.

Late in the evening there was a call for Mrs. B. It was the lady at one of her new homes. She was having trouble with a resident. Mrs. B. gave her advice based on experience: (1) "If a guy can dial a number, knows who his guardian is, and knows when he gets a paycheck, he's got a lot on the ball, honey." (2) "Don't let residents compare us with other homes as a means of manipulating us. Empha-size that we are taking as good care of them as we can." (3) "Sit down and visit with him. Have a cup of coffee and learn more about him. That will help."

Again I was struck by Mrs. B's spontaneous, yet proper, response. Her advice reflected (1) expectations and recognition of competence, (2) awareness of manipulative tactics, and (3) learning from the resi-dent rather than setting rigid, punitive limits.

Mrs. B. thanked me for calling her to the phone each time I did so. Jim asked her about joining a health club that costs $80 a year. She asked him to contact his guardian directly. When he hesitated, she offered to place the call for him but he'd have to talk to the guardian himself. Thus she skillfully pushed him to the strongest effort he was willing and able to put forth, and the result was a success. His guardian agreed to pay the fee for the club.

Many expressions like "Beautiful!" and "Very good!" are used in this setting. Verbal, sincere praise and sharing of good feelings reinforce both normative behavior and the social ties that help make the behavior meaningful.

Mrs. B. asked if I was feeling better and smiled when I said "Yes." She asked me to speak up about my likes and dislikes because otherwise they wouldn't know what my preferences were. She was in and out this morning, watering the lawn, doing dishes, and cleaning upstairs.

R. came in complaining of insomnia. Mrs. B. advised him to find something else to do when he can't sleep, such as writing a letter or reading. "You can always call me anytime at night. You have my phone number."

November 21

At 11:00 A.M. there was a phone call for me from Dr. Farberow informing me that Mrs. B., suspicious of my identity, had checked my story by phoning to Florida and calling the VA regional office. She had uncovered discrepancies. We arranged a meeting with my social worker. After considering various possibilities and contingencies we decided to abort this phase of the project. We met with Mrs. B. and explained to her the nature and purpose of the project.

L HOME DEBRIEFING

Although there is the possibility of a leak in security, here we simply point out the aspects of our presentation which made Mrs. B. suspicious of David Kent's identity. It is noteworthy that Mrs. B. is a registered nurse, a former plainclothes policewoman, an experienced family-care manager, and a sharply intuitive woman.

The following practical items may have aroused Mrs. B.'s suspicions about David Kent's identity. (1) The medication (25 mg of Elavil twice a day) seemed very low. (In fact, a daily intake of 50 mg of Elavil is an adequate maintenance dose, according to Dr. Crockett.) (2) Suicidal persons are not usually allowed the privilege of self-medication. Obviously, Mrs. B. expected to see a much sicker person than David Kent seemed to be. (3) The referral information sheet was not so complete for Kent as it was for other residents. (The social worker disagreed on this point.)

As to David Kent's behavior, Mrs. B. found him to be too polite, too steady in handwriting, too careful in his eating habits, too alert, and too willing to take medication to be accepted as a bona fide suicidal patient. We think these qualities are consistent with a somewhat compulsive "dependent-satisfied" person who reacts to rejection and abandonment with depression and suicide attempts. It may well be that Mrs. B. reacted to other, subtler cues that signaled artificiality, but she was unable to bring them to awareness and communicate them when pressured to provide intellectualized rationales for her intuition.

At any rate, Mrs. B.'s suspicions led her to check the Florida background data by a long-distance phone call and to investigate Kent's C-file numbers with the VA regional office. Her doubts fully aroused, she contacted the social worker, believing that the hospital had planted someone without his knowledge or that of the ward staff. Keith was in an awkward position. He was unwilling to deceive Mrs. B. further when she asked him directly to check on Kent's story. Putting her off for the moment, he got hold of Dr. Farberow who, in turn, called David Kent and set up the subsequent meeting.

Mrs. B.'s protectiveness led her to decide it was best for us to withhold revelation of the research to her resident guests. An informal friendship between the senior author and Mrs. B. continued after completion of the project. There were gift exchanges at Christmastime, attendance at her son's confirmation later that year, and occasional visits and telephone calls.

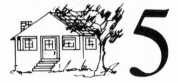 **5**

W HOME

Our next choice for a research setting, Mrs. G.'s family-care home, proved to be unavailable. Mrs. G. already had one suicidal resident and felt that a second one would give her too much responsibility.

Continuing our selection from the list of managers who had agreed to accept a researcher as resident, we contacted Mrs. W. She said she would take Kent. She wanted him to come for Thanksgiving dinner and did, in fact, hold dinner until he arrived. Mrs. W., a buxom black woman who was nearly sixty years old, was under treatment for hypertension. As a former nurse, she was familiar with health care from both consumer and provider points of view. She was a devout Christian and a regular churchgoer.

Mrs. W.'s home was described by social workers as a modest but well-furnished one-story house with a homey atmosphere. It has one single and one double bedroom for residents. It is near a shopping center, churches, and a recreation center. The sponsor is an elderly widow and a retired LVN. A pleasant, motherly person, she seems to have a keen sense of responsibility. She worked for many years in a Los Angeles hospital. She has an interest in helping people and at the same time wants to augment her retirement income. The social workers believed that quiet middle-aged or elderly veterans would be appropriate for W Home.

KENT'S W HOME JOURNAL

November 24

Mrs. W. speaks in a low, gravelly voice. She is an elderly black woman, a nurse. Miss English, a stand-in social worker, said she would like to look around because this was her first visit to W

Home. Mrs. W. was going to take only the social worker on a tour, but Miss English suggested that I go along.

The home is well kept up and quite clean. It is located in a lower middle-class black neighborhood not far from a community college. At present there seem to be only two other residents, both black. Mrs. W. lives in a small unit at the rear which is separate from the house but accessible by an intercom system.

She talked briefly with me, asking what I liked to do. "Do you like to watch TV?" She said they had saved dinner for me. It was 2:45 in the afternoon. I sat on the couch with my suitcase and a cardboard box. Mrs. W. asked Miss English to come into the kitchen for a talk.

Mrs. W. and J. moved some things out of a room so that I could move in. Then Mrs. W. picked up my box, led me to the room, and started putting things away for me. I began helping and she went off to fix dinner.

We ate at 3:00 P.M. Since I wasn't very hungry, I ate only a little. The meal was served family style to the three of us residents at the dining room table. H. carefully clasped his hands and prayed before eating. J., my roommate, is very polite to Mrs. W.; in fact, with his many "Ma'ams," he is almost obsequious. She has more or less turned me over to him. For example, at the table she told him to ask me if I smoked. J. praised Mrs. W.'s cooking, and indeed the food was quite good.

After a few minutes I went in to lie down on my bed. I heard Mrs. W. telling the guys that David must be tired. She relayed some of the information from my social service referral form: he surely is meek; he tried to kill himself once. She felt they should try to get me to talk and go out some. She mistakenly told J. I had a wife in Pittsburgh (not Saint Petersburg). Then I fell asleep for an hour.

Putting away my things took a lot of time. For a while I just sat looking at the suitcase. Getting settled seemed like an overwhelming task.

I went into the living room to read. The only good reading lamps are there. J. sat dozing in a nearby armchair. Mrs. W. came in and made small talk. She told me I look like B., a former resident. She asked what book I was reading, what branch of the service I had been in, whether or not I was hurt in service, when I was in, and so forth. I answered with nods and soft sounds. She said I am supposed to try to talk more. J. is a good talker, she noted, and they laughed together about it.

She served pie to J. and H. about 5:15 P.M. I said I wasn't very hungry. Later she showed me the procedures for paying. She took me back to her little house, gave me a business card, carefully counted my money and change a second time, and gave me a receipt, explaining then that I would pay rent on the 24th of each month. She brought me back to the main house and turned me over to J., explaining I was to take medication with him at 9 A.M. and 9 P.M. I was told to feel free to call her anytime.

As she left Mrs. W. told J., almost sarcastically, "I know you're going to have a good night." They laughed. I know I'm a drag to have around. But why are they putting me on with these double meanings? It's as if they're conspirators to make life superficially acceptable but at the same time denying me real closeness. At this point, however, I don't care much about closeness anyway.

I read and watched TV and dozed. I had to borrow J.'s *TV Guide.* He's kind and big-brotherly, a bit slow but steady. I forgot to turn off the TV, but he did it for me. We took medications together.

I showered and wrote these notes in the bathroom.

November 25

At 6:45 A.M. J. was quietly moving about the room. I waited under the cover until he went back to bed. I felt unable to handle a good-morning routine. But when I got up J. did, too, in order to show me which towel and washcloth were mine. (I had used his last night.) I washed up and went into the living room to read.

Sounds are important to me. This house is located near a jet landing pattern with the occasional unnerving roar. There is soothing stereo music coming over the intercom from early morning until night. The street sounds and the voices of children at play reinforce my feeling of isolation. J.'s clock ticks loudly all night near my ear.

Mrs. W. came in about 7:30 A.M. and began to prepare breakfast. She called good-morning to me in her friendly, yet distant, voice. At 7:55 she awoke H. and J. and called us to breakfast. "Do you like oatmeal, David?" she asked. I nodded.

Again I ate only a little. What's the use of eating? Eating implies a future; it provides energy for later. Who cares about my "later"? The other fellows had eggs, sausage, and toast. Mrs. W. asked if I wanted sausage, too. I shook my head. She told me that here we take our dishes into the kitchen, rinse them, and set them on the drainboard. I did it in two trips, rinsing even the unused glass and silverware. Then I went to bed.

At 8:30 A.M. Mrs. W. woke me up to show me where she'd placed my cup with one pill in it. She told me to take it at 9 o'clock. Then she left. J. and H. were in bed asleep. I wrote again in the bathroom. My pill was still in the cup. It was 9:45 A.M. I "took" my medication and thus had two pills in my pocket. I watched football on TV while J. and H. slept. Mrs. W. came in again and said, "Hello." Then she began bustling about in the kitchen.

Pork chops, French fried potatoes, and tomato salad were served at 12:45 P.M. There wasn't much on my plate (e.g., one pork chop compared with H.'s three), for she had anticipated my small appetite.

I watched football for a while and then went to bed and read.

I had the feeling that as long as I didn't cause any trouble I'd be allowed to stay here forever and keep to myself. Compared with the large impersonal board-and-care homes, this place has better furnishings and tastier home cooking. Disadvantages include a lack of space in which to move around and fewer possibilities of finding someone who is compatible and available for interaction. Since there were only three names to learn, I knew them already. Oh, yes, there are two cats.

I stood in the doorway watching kids playing outside in the street. I had to get up and move around. Sitting or lying down for prolonged periods produces a heavy-headed, headachy feeling. The house is very warm, and the contrast between very dark and very light areas makes my eyes tire quickly while reading or watching TV. The sheer physiological shake-up that accompanies depressives' sedentary existence complicates the symptom pattern. I'm convinced that some depressives would feel better if they were encouraged to move about.

J. went out after lunch, returning at 7 P.M. H. stayed in his room until Mrs. W. called the two of us at 4:30 P.M. for pie and ice cream. H. praised Mrs. W. for the dessert, perhaps too effusively. The pattern here seems to be two meals a day plus dessert in the evening. Cultural or convenient?

I'm glad I was in another family-care unit with a black sponsor because otherwise I would worry that my feeling so distant from Mrs. W. is predominantly a cultural and racial reaction. I did not feel the same way with Mrs. B., who is also black.

Mrs. W. leaves as soon as she has served us a meal. Because we empty our plates and rinse them, she has no way of knowing whether or not we ate unless she asks and we reply truthfully. Her apparent lack of interest in us contrasts sharply with Mrs. B.'s concern for her residents. Mrs. B. used her awareness of my not eating to express caring and nurturance.

More television. J. came out of the bedroom, and from 8 to 9 P.M. he dozed and watched TV, too. Then he went to bed without reminding me of my medication. He doesn't seem to care either.

I went to bed at 11 o'clock without taking a shower. Why should I bother?

November 26

While J. and Mrs. W. were gone in the car, I walked to a mailbox and sent off a set of notes. The neighborhood seems monotonous. No entertainment, few stores.

Back to the television set. Mrs. W. came in about 9:30 A.M., reminded me of my pill, gave me a new *TV Guide,* and told me she was going to church. She didn't ask me if I wanted to go with her, even though she had invited me the day before.

I was alone (H. was in his room, as usual). At 1:15 P.M. I wandered into the kitchen. On the cupboard was an open package of rat poison. It seemed to be an invitation. What would she do if I took some? Would she care? Apparently Mrs. W. doesn't see me as a suicide risk. The circumstance tempts me to make a suicidal gesture, but I'm not angry enough (yet) to make a serious attempt. The anger is still minimal because no one here promises more than he or she cares enough to deliver. Obviously, Mrs. W. thinks she is doing what is necessary by providing a new, clean house and meals. Her other two residents seem satisfied; anyway, they praise her efforts. But at this point I've already decided to leave. There's little to be learned in terms of research by staying longer than a week, for the pattern has already emerged. And David Kent would rather go back to the hospital than wither away here. Perhaps a social worker can pick me up on Thursday.

Mrs. W. returned about 1:45 P.M. She got home "early" from church this Sunday. She listened to gospel programs on the radio as she puttered in the kitchen. We ate TV dinners, beets, and peaches at about 2:15. TV dinners followed by TV! Is it boring for the reader to read of television, television, television? It is boring to live that way, too.

Mrs. W. brought ice cream to my chair this evening, saying that I could eat it there. H. got to eat his in his room. This house is a cupboard for storing people. A twilight place for living. Or is it really "living"?

"Have a good night. Call me if you need me," said Mrs. W., and she was gone again. I wonder if she knows what Kent expects from her or needs from her? By Tuesday he's going to begin having thoughts of killing himself which will necessitate calling his social worker to take him back to the hospital on Thursday. Partly it's planned; partly it's inevitable. It will seem abrupt to Mrs. W. in much the same way that acts seem abrupt in hospital records because staff members haven't sensed the precursors to action.

I wrote notes at 6:10 P.M. J. is still gone. How senselessly we worried about note writing before I entered this setting! There is little else but privacy and opportunity to write.

Interestingly, as my life again narrowed and became more simple I found myself deeply moved by maudlin TV shows, just as I was emotionally affected by movies in the psychiatric hospital. Similarly, washing, brushing my teeth, and exercising take on more importance and receive more attention than they do in my other, busy life. My world has shrunk in about me and much of my attention is directed inward, since outer stimuli are dull and repetitious or even nonexistent. Tomorrow I really must go outside for a walk, I thought. As for tonight — well, I went back to watching TV. The set is always waiting to help erase time.

November 27

Mrs. W. informed me that she would take me to see a nearby college later that morning. J. asked if I was going to enroll there. As Mrs. W. seemed doubtful, I felt doubtful, too. She told J. that we were going so that, when Keith (my other social worker) called, we could say we'd been to see the college. Mrs. W. asked J. about his weekend. He said he got back about 9 o'clock last night, but it was actually later than that. She didn't exactly call him on it, but she said she was up listening to the radio at that time and wondering if he was back.

As J. left I said good-bye to him. He seemed surprised and pleased. He stopped and told me he was going to the mental hygiene clinic and would be back later. The appointment card on his dresser indicated a 10:15 A.M. appointment, but he had to leave before 8 o'clock because of difficult bus connections.

H. had received some information about training in tax assessing and was considering taking the course. Mrs. W. obviously felt that this plan was unrealistic. She asked skeptically if he was good with figures. She laughed off the idea, ending the conversation with the offhand remark, "Keep on trying." H., suppressing any hostility he felt about her put-down, thanked her with the overpoliteness that marks his dealings, and J.'s, with Mrs. W. Both men are models of considerateness, politeness, and minding their own business. I wonder what they do with anger.

Mrs. W. offered to fix another pancake for me as she served another to H., but I refused. The offer was important, for the little signs of kindness and personal interest shown me this morning had a big impact on my outlook. I was so starved for displays of concern that I felt warm and cared about for the moment.

Mrs. W. came in about 9:30 A.M. She said I looked very good in the outfit I was wearing. She put some clothes in the washer and then showed me where to put mine for her to wash. Then she explained and demonstrated how to make my bed. She bustled around emptying wastebaskets and putting my suitcase away.

Finally, she ushered me out to her car for our trip to the local college. We saw H. on the way and gave him a ride. "He goes walking every day — he's obese," she explained. She gave me directions concerning the route as she drove. At the college we stopped; H. waited in the car while Mrs. W. and I walked through a couple of buildings. Then we drove around the perimeter of the campus, Mrs. W. pointing out the administration building where I'd register. In fact, she read aloud almost every sign in sight (trying to be helpful, I suppose, but implying that I couldn't read for myself), even noting the children and dogs in the yards of nearby campus housing as if explaining to a child.

When we got back I said I wanted to go for a walk. Mrs. W. checked to see if I had her business card. She pointed out an important geographic reference point on the corner of our block, a church I hadn't noticed before. She didn't want me to get lost.

I was wrong about this area being uninteresting. The new direction in which we traveled this morning revealed numerous shops of all kinds. Since I have become sensitive to food (and its lack) in this setting, I noticed several restaurants, markets, and snack bars. On my walk I bought snacks to take back with me.

I appreciate the anonymity of the consumer role. I enjoy being called "Sir," knowing then that I don't look very different from other customers in the stores. This area is a better location for family-care units than an elegant neighborhood, where being a bit strange would make salespeople notice an ex-patient and perhaps make him feel awkward.

Coming back after an hour's walk, I met Mrs. W. in the kitchen as she was finishing up the clothes. She asked where I'd been. I told her I'd walked to the college and got lost coming back (both true). She laughed and said that that's the best way to learn. I went to bed for about an hour; it was tiring to walk after even a few days of inactivity.

Later that afternoon I went for another walk. It was a warm, smoggy day in Los Angeles. I passed J. returning on the other side of the street. He called and I waved. I ate an eclair and bought some gum at a market.

Walking back, I noticed that the house in which we lived was rather drab and that the fence was in need of paint. Mrs. W. called to me from her cottage as I walked through the back gate. She was chatting with J. She invited me to sit down and asked where I'd been. I offered them some gum. She was glad I was back because she didn't want to get in her car to go looking for me after dark. She didn't really expect much of me. She asked, "You're not hungry, are you?" I shook my head. I said I'd better go lie down. It makes me tired to walk.

About 5:30 P.M. she asked if I wanted ice cream. Soon H. and I had ice cream while J. ate his dinner, saved from 1:15 P.M. Mrs. W. said that J. had bought a *TV Guide* this week, I should buy one next week, and (she laughed) H. should buy one after that. "Yes, Mrs. W.," said H. "That's right, Mrs. W." As usual Mrs. W. disappeared after serving us.

Afterward H. came out of his room into J.'s and mine to borrow a cigarette. It takes a pretty strong desire to get H. out of his room to interact. Mrs. W. strictly regulates his smoking.

I'm increasingly concerned about the ways in which life in this house is structured for the convenience of Mrs. W. Although somewhat interested in us, she is much more concerned to present a good front and to keep her routine and her privacy intact. She's likeable in her way and certainly not malicious, but she is perhaps unable and certainly unmotivated to do more than she is now doing.

We watched football on television. J. left when the game started.

I think that's his way of avoiding conflicts. He bought the *TV Guide* but handed it to me, saying, "I don't use it much." Appeasement and politeness are his tactics. Again, I wonder how he handles unavoidable anger. H. watched the entire game; he knew what teams were playing, and he seemed alert to the game's progress. When it was over, I "took" my medication and went to bed.

November 28

I sat, simply sat, in the new chair in our room for half an hour until Mrs. W. came in to call us to breakfast. "Oh, you're just sitting in the chair," she commented, but she didn't seem to worry about the implications of my changed behavior. Breakfast consisted of orange juice, milk, and three pancakes; the others had more pancakes and also sausages. I was served less probably because several days earlier I had eaten only part of my food. My appetite has improved, but Mrs. W. hasn't adapted to the change, nor can she check on it, because of our food disposal routine. I feel discriminated against, and the irrational but immediate thought is that it's because I'm white and Mrs. W. doesn't really like me.

I went for a long walk shortly before 9 A.M. (Mrs. W. said she would give me my pill after I returned.) She warned me to keep only about fifty cents with me when I went out. Another resident walking outside had his wallet stolen and then had nothing. "We don't steal here [in the house]," she said, so it's safe to leave money there. I believe her.

As I started out a mongrel dog that was part husky raced toward me as if to attack me. Thoroughly startled and shaking a bit, I continued on my walk anyway. It was the first rush of adrenalin in my system in quite a while, and I overreacted to it. Many people in this neighborhood have big barking dogs for protection. I wandered about aimlessly, looking in shop windows.

My time sense is changing again. When one has all day to do only a few things, he can begin them at leisure and string them out as long as it's comfortable to do so. Time becomes not a limiting factor to be outwitted but a resource to be used at one's whim.

I recall a dream I had a couple of nights ago. It was another of the fear-of-becoming-insane sort. I dreamed that I looked out over a field with rocks, plants, and people in it. In the dream I "knew" that if I could see these elements with Zen-like objectivity, without attaching value to one over the other, I would be omniscient — but also insane. My mind started to move toward viewing everything dispassionately and then I became frightened, retreated, and moved on to other dream material without waking.

I mailed off another batch of notes and walked several miles before returning. I thought I saw condescending and contemptuous smiles on the faces of some passersby on the street.

J. has been in bed all day (except for meals). It's no wonder he tosses and smokes at night. I told him I didn't expect to be here long since I was beginning to have thoughts about hurting myself. He sat forward in his chair and asked me to repeat myself. I did. "Oh," he said.

In the morning, as I sat reading, Mrs. W. came in to fix breakfast. I told her I wasn't feeling at all well. "Don't feel that way; life is beautiful," she said. A few minutes later she continued, "Would you like to talk to me later? Sometimes that helps." I didn't know if anything would help. She added, "After J. goes to work we'll go for a little ride. I'll take you with me."

Mrs. W. dropped J. off at work. H. muttered longingly about his wish to have a job like that. Then he and Mrs. W. engaged in colorless conversation about the weather, the sky, the streets we were passing, and the traffic as we drove up the freeway to visit a friend whose father had just died in Louisiana. She parked the car, and H. and I waited in it for ten minutes while she went inside the house to "pay her respects." She asked if we had enjoyed the ride. "I sure did, Mrs. W. Thank-you, Mrs. W.," H. replied effusively.

About 9:30 A.M. Mrs. W. called me over to the table. She had some information forms to fill out on me. Noticeable among the items were questions about next of kin. I guess she wanted to know whom to contact if I should commit suicide. She gave me a sheet to sign, presenting me with the back of the form where the signature goes. I hesitated. "Just sign here," she said. I started to turn it over to read it. I asked her whether I would get some money back if I left before a month was up. She assured me that I would. So I went ahead and signed without reading the form. That satisfied her. I guess she thought I wouldn't understand much of it anyway. Again, she doesn't expect much of us. I keep repeating this observation — the pressure toward incompetence is constant.

She took me outside into a little patio area where we began to talk about my problem. I told her I thought I might be going back to the hospital soon, that I was having self-destructive thoughts, that perhaps "they" had let me out too soon, and that maybe my medication wasn't strong enough. She insisted that I had to give myself a chance. She said that I'm good looking and still young; I could go to school (take one class at first if I felt like it) and perhaps find a girl friend there. "Life is everything" she told me, adding that if I jumped into the water I'd *have* to swim. "Then you could be the kind of man you've always wanted to be," she continued. "We can't be happy all the time but we've got to be tough." If I needed anything (Did I drink coffee? she asked suddenly? perhaps she thought that was my problem), I should just let her know. And I should talk to her anytime I needed to.

About that time my social worker called from the VA. Mrs. W. told him we had just been talking about him, and then she relayed to him the general sense of what she had been telling me. He asked to talk to me. She discreetly stayed out of sight (and out of earshot for part of the time) while he and I talked. He arranged for me to call him back from a public phone later that morning.

Soon I told Mrs. W. I wanted to go for a walk. She praised me for getting out on my own. While I was out I called Keith back and made arrangements for my next placement. As I walked home, a black man sitting on his porch shouted at me, "I told you to keep that head up!" Then, soothingly, "You'll feel better." It startled and stung me to find my depression so visible, even to strangers. He could toy with me at will.

On my return Mrs. W. called me to sit with her in the patio. Already today we had enjoyed more interaction than in all the preceding five days. She asked where I had been and what I had done, expressing interest and pleasure in my activities. This rather sudden expression of personal concern was rather less effective than it would have been if she had started out that way. She groped for topics to keep the conversation going — my ward number, the make of car I used to drive, my driver's license, even my watch manufacturer. She asked her usual, "Do you like _____ ?" This time it was, "Do you like sliced tomatoes? We're having them for lunch." I nodded, as usual. She asked, "Are you hungry?" I replied, "Not very; I'm never very hungry anymore." She told me that's why she doesn't put as much on my plate as she gives the other residents, but there's always plenty of food. If I'm hungry, I must tell her so.

In general, Mrs. W. and the staff at the larger board-and-care facilities in which I lived are predominately reactive in their relationships with residents. If there is an obvious problem, particularly if the resident comes to them with it, they respond conscientiously. Mrs. B., on the other hand, is active in her relationship with her residents, seeking them out and deliberately involving them in her life. A reactive attitude may mean that concrete help and demonstrations of caring are too late for the withdrawn suicidal ex-patient.

Another difference between Mrs. B. and Mrs. W. is that the former immediately brought the issue of race to the surface, recognizing its existence but demonstrating (as well as telling me) that it's less important than the personal relationship between two people. The racial differences in this neighborhood and in W Home flicker just below the surface, causing unnecessary misunderstandings.

Mrs. W. promised to take us for a ride this afternoon after 2 o'clock. (She watches TV shows from 1 to 2 P.M.) She tried, also, to get me to promise to visit her church and to go to a Christmas party there on December 14. But she's lost me already, and I think she knows it. I wonder if she knows why. I doubt it.

Shortly after 2 o'clock Mrs. W. called H. and me to go for a ride. She had taken seriously H.'s suggestion that high-test gasoline might alleviate the ping in her car, so on the way to the butcher's we stopped and got some. She asked if we wanted to go in with her while she shopped. We did. She asked if I had chewed all the gum I'd bought the other day because she never sees me chewing it.

After we returned I headed for bed. She closed the front door as she said, "I don't want you to catch cold." I'm glad she cares, but I've been blowing my nose for a week with a cold. Too late, too late.

We had TV dinners, unexpectedly, at 4:20 P.M. It's hard to predict when and what we'll eat. Again it was for her convenience that we ate at that hour, for at 5:15 she was to go with friends to visit someone in the hospital. I finally opened a conversation with H. at the table. This is the first day since he's been here (three months) that he's taken two rides in one day. Rides are relatively rare. He walks and sleeps to pass time. He remarked that he doesn't always get enough to eat, but he thanks Mrs. W. profusely at every meal. He does seem to like her. The other two residents who have been here during his stay went out "to some place bigger." They were both blacks. I wonder if I'm the first Caucasian to live here. I asked H. if people bother him when he goes walking. He said that they don't.

November 30

When I came back from a walk at noon, Mrs. W. asked me where I'd gone. I told her. She asked if I had seen the movie theaters along my way, and she offered to take me to a movie anytime I liked. Maybe she thinks I'm going to stay; she certainly talks as though she thinks so. I went to bed.

Soon thereafter we had a delicious chicken dinner. Later I noticed Mrs. W. icing a chocolate cake. Things are picking up now that I'm going.

Interestingly, what I covet is the hour from 1 to 2 P.M. which Mrs. W. reserves for herself, as well as the general privacy she maintains. The depressed person, with his immaturity and his self-doubting, may be very perceptive in picking out the aspects of life we hold to be our own and then demanding them of us as expressions of our concern for him. He believes that only the sacrifice of our most precious possessions can express his worth in our eyes.

Why is it that people try to respond to another's depression with attempts to cheer him, with excessive hopefulness and cheerfulness? When he fails to respond or rejects them, they may feel anger or abandonment, or both. When he accepts their efforts and advice but cannot change his mood, there may be pity or disdain. Why can't people accept his sadness, honor it, and try to share it with him through empathy?

After supper I said to J., "I wonder what rat poison tastes like." "What?" he asked. I repeated my comment and added, "There's some over there." "Oh, I don't know," he said. I doubt that he picked anything up from the exchange or that he'll relay the conversation to Mrs. W.

Talking about poison brings up another issue: Why don't we train patients and residents in suicide prevention? They would get more cues from their fellows than from any other role group, simply because they spend more time together. I'd like to see training programs in therapy in general and suicide prevention in particular for the patients themselves. Such programs would have a worthwhile result in injecting trained mental health workers into the community, where they could be a leavening agent. It is better for patients to be workers than to be worked on by others.

J. and I watched TV in the evening. We have an arrangement now, checking on our preferences in programs. J. left to go to the store for a few minutes. Before going he asked if there was anything I wanted. It was a small but important gesture.

I started packing unobtrusively, I'm looking forward to my next setting.

December 1

After breakfast, when Mrs. W. had returned from the fish market with catfish, she and J. (still in his pajamas, as usual) talked for half an hour in the kitchen. She was making another chocolate cake. They laughed about H.'s getting fatter and fatter. Mrs. W. said, "Poor soul! I guess we have only one life to live." They know H. enjoys eating. Then, in lowered tones, they talked about my social worker, who is coming today, and about me. From my chair in the living room I couldn't hear this part of the conversation. The talk turned to various television programs. Then J. went back to bed.

H. came out of his room at about 8:40 and headed for his morning walk. He conversed with Mrs. W. for a few minutes, telling her, as usual, what a wonderful woman she is and how no one works for us as she does. He went on and on. Obviously Mrs. W. has often heard this kind of talk from H., but she told him that it makes her feel good. She said she tries to treat people the way she would want to be treated. H. is looking forward to enjoying some of that chocolate cake, but his feelings of affection and gratitude are genuine. I sensed a tone of overplaying, of "putting on," in their voices, but I don't know if that's the cultural style for praise here.

Keith arrived shortly before noon. He and Mrs. W. were talking about me in the living room as I came out of the bathroom. Mrs. W. was telling him she thought it might be the money that was motivating me to go back to the hospital. (Keith later expressed the possibility that her comment may have been an indirect reference to the racial-cultural differences.) I'm still fascinated by the idea that people seem to expect a mental patient to hear what is said only when they talk directly to him.

I walked into the living room. Mrs. W. went into the kitchen so that my social worker and I could talk. Keith asked me how I was doing. I told him that everyone was kind here, but I didn't think I had been ready to leave the hospital. I explained that I shudder each time I pass the rat poison and that the medication isn't strong enough.

He agreed that I should go back to the hospital. He told me to get my things together while he took care of the financial details. It was a relief to let him take the responsibility for telling Mrs. W. of our decision and getting my refund. He later told me she had the money (in cash) ready in a marked envelope. She knew that I had begun packing the night before (she must have checked my dresser drawers when I took my walk). I had been given no key so there was no key to return.

As we left J. and Mrs. W. shook my hand and wished me good luck. H. was out walking.

W HOME DEBRIEFING

December 22

Mrs. W.: David Kent was quiet but kept active; he wanted to go to Pepperdine.

He was afraid to go to school so I told him he didn't have to carry a heavy load but could begin with just one or two subjects. Then, if he did well, he could advance to whatever level he could manage. He hadn't stayed here long enough for us to do much of anything. Very nice, very quiet, and very cooperative. One morning he said he didn't feel well. I said, "What's the matter?" He said he was having those same thoughts again. I said, "Oh, no!" you know, trying to cheer him up.

J: I knew you were a little different from other people I've met. I thought you were nice and intelligent.

DKR suggested that Mrs. W. might check sometimes before dishes are scraped and rinsed to see how much food has been eaten.

Mrs. W.: I used to sit with them. Then it seemed as if they resented it. So to give 'em a free hand I would disappear so they could feel free to say what they wanted to about me, whether it was good or bad. I feel that as long as you eat, I don't care how much you eat — you just eat till it's gone. That's what I told David. David didn't eat all I had prepared for him. Well, I never remonstrated with him for that; if they don't want to eat, it's OK. But I won't give them more the next time and, I tell them, not so much "because you didn't eat everything the last time." And I feel that I'd rather they wanted more than to give 'em more and have 'em throw it away.

DKR spoke about the rat poison.

Mrs. W. said she believes she corrected that problem by putting a napkin over the poison.

DKR: Have you had white residents before?

Mrs. W.: There was a white man here who planned to go to Pepperdine; his doctor was nearby so this place was ideal for him. He stayed until he got ill and he passed away. And that was about two and a half years.

DKR: Did you feel uncomfortable with me because I am white? [No one had expressed any discomfort.]

Mrs. W. distinguished between here and the South. And in the South she distinguished between those you know [on the basis of personal acquaintance] and those you don't know.

DKR expressed interest in the form he had signed.

Mrs. W.: You know what? And I said to myself, "David, don't leave." But I didn't, you know, I couldn't tell him. You can't keep people if they don't want to stay. And I was wondering what I had done . . . and I said I think I was very nice to him. I brought in the sheet, and he said, "If I go back to the hospital, will my money be refunded?" And I said, "Sure." And I didn't think he would leave. [She wondered how DK could tell in only a week — she hoped he would give it a chance. In a month or so he would "have a better feeling, pro or con, about me."]

J. mentioned that the last time they went to the VA hospital Mrs. W. said, "I wonder where David is?"

NLF: It sounds as if you really got to like David.

Mrs. W.: I did, you know, and it looked to me as if I was really trying hard to let him know that I wanted him to stay. But I didn't want to go overboard. At that time I had two cats, and I said, "Are you interested in the cats?" But, you know, he wasn't interested. We visited, and I told him that if he needed me, just to let me know.

DKR wondered about mealtimes and the two-meal system. He suggested that the purpose of the system be explained to new residents.

Mrs. W.: I didn't want my guests going to bed on a heavy meal. If I served a big midday meal, the residents had time to walk it off. I also served a big breakfast, country style. I don't want to shirk my duties, you know. So I feel that if my people are fed, they don't care where I am as long as they're content. [In the hospital the heaviest meal is at noon, she asserted from her nursing experience. She agreed that explaining the meal system to a newcomer would be a good idea.]

NLF asked if she felt it would be useful to have more information about residents when they arrive and, if so, what kind.

Mrs. W. had never got a write-up on H. because he had been referred from another board-and-care place. The hospital follow-up on DK was the first one Mrs. W. has had. She has no information about H.'s hospitalization or symptoms. She said, "Now I had this room and I would have given it to him [DK], but the green sheet said to encourage him to have conversation so I put him in with J." She was a bit saddened that DK was intelligent but wasn't going to give Pepperdine College a try. She felt sorry for him and Sharon for getting divorced so young. There was a resident who had a wife named Sharon, and J.'s daughter was named Sharon. "I'm glad you turned out to be what you are 'cause my impression of you was that you had a bleak future." She wished that Kent had already achieved an education: "If they don't get it while they're young. it's kind of hard to get it when they're older." She recalled that he hadn't quite earned his Associate of Arts degree.

DKR asked how the Christmas party went.

Mrs. W.: Oh, beautiful. I missed you. I was looking for you. Each resident got a present and food, and there was square dancing. It was at a Catholic center on East Boulevard. You had the whole hall to yourself. There was a resident who played the piano and the group sang Christmas carols. I just had a ball!

NLF thanked everybody for the interchange of information and perspectives.

DKR informed the people from W Home that our policy is to keep the research settings anonymous in our presentations and that we would offer a general summary of our study at the sponsors' meeting in the spring.

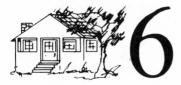6 S MANOR

The final aftercare setting for our experiential research was S Manor. It is the least structured of the four in terms of programs and supervision. Set in a middle-class white neighborhood, the buildings that compose S Manor blend in with the surrounding apartment houses.

A social worker described it as "a four-unit apartment building with three bedrooms and one bathroom in each unit. There is a separate central dining room. Meals are provided. The location is near a hospital and is convenient to all shopping facilities and to bus lines. This facility is suitable for veterans who function fairly well and with a minimum of supervision."

Like many of his peers, David Randolph (a new pseudonym) had become something of a connoisseur of residential aftercare facilities by the time he was placed in S Manor. There was expected overlap but this living place also had unique aspects.

S MANOR JOURNAL

Friday, December 1

We arrived just before 2:00 P.M. Suitcase in hand, I followed my social worker into a yard where a young man and a big dog were standing. The man was watering the lawn. He and his wife (JD and FD), the managers, were greeted by my social worker. The lady was very businesslike and quickly took charge. She signed me in and gave me a receipt for two weeks' rent. She didn't have the necessary ninety-five cents change. I assumed she would get it to me later. After giving me a key she took us up to the room and introduced me to one of my two roommates. She told me to come down in a few minutes so she could show me the dining room and introduce me to someone with whom I could ride the bus to my VA job on Monday. Then I unpacked.

My roommate told me that at 2 P.M. there would be a coffee break, but I wasn't interested. He went out. Soon I went down to the managers' house. F. gave me an information sheet and took me to the TV room where I met the resident who would guide me to the VA on Monday morning. "David is from your ward, 210," she said. She asked the resident to take me across the street to the dining room, as she herself was busy now.

The resident complied, introducing me to the cook as "the new member." My roommate was sitting there with a cup of coffee. Back in the TV room there was a good selection of paperback books, a cribbage board, puzzles, games, magazines, and a TV set, as well as game tables and chairs.

I nearly forgot where my room was. Luckily, I found it. I had already forgotten the names of everyone who had been introduced to me. At 2:40 P.M. my roommate came in to watch TV. He volunteered information about the hours of meals. He seemed friendly and helpful, but I only wanted to lie down and rest. I was so very tired.

I felt rather experienced at adjusting to new living accommodations. This room was rather good. There was plenty of drawer space and sufficient closets and cupboards. The framed pictures on the wall were pleasing. Furnishings were good; sheets were clean; heating was adequate; and my roommates weren't obviously different from two guys you might live with in a dormitory or in navy barracks. The atmosphere was relatively hopeful for David Randolph.

I went to the bathroom to learn where it was and what it was like. The trip also seemed to be a primitive kind of settling-in behavior.

People here seem more "together" and younger than those at B Home. In the TV room that evening one of the residents volunteered to go out to buy soft drinks for several others who were watching TV. Another group of residents were planning to go for a walk. A third group of three or four left for a movie. Obviously, the "coalition" (Reynolds and Farberow, 1976) among residents is strong here. There is a good, healthy esprit de corps.

Saturday, December 2

After breakfast I dozed off, then heard the cleaning ladies come into the room. There was something in the information sheet about getting out of bed and out of the room while they cleaned, so I started to get up. "Lay back down. I don't care," the older woman said. They vacuumed, emptied wastebaskets, and cleaned the bathroom. One roommate went out but the other, like me, stayed in bed. At 9:30 we made a fine pair: one was sitting up in bed, half asleep; the other was snoring, having gotten up only to eat.

Later I watched football on TV in the lounge downstairs. A quick way of assessing the level of regression of residents in a facility might be to check on the kinds of TV programs they watch. Cartoons and old Western reruns are turned on relatively infrequently here. Last night there was news on and today two football games were watched. There are also more comments and conversations in the lounge than at the other facilities in which I've stayed. Some residents are disturbed, to be sure, but many others show no apparent disturbances.

There was talk of a picnic today. Some guys left. I felt left out, increasingly so today as people seemed to ignore me. I received no greetings at all. Again, we should think carefully about the day of the week on which we place a person in an aftercare setting. Weekends can be very dull and lonely. Perhaps suicides in aftercare facilities occur more frequently on Saturdays, Sundays, and Mondays than on other days.

I went to lunch (beans and franks) at noon. As usual, the day's menu (listing the main course only and signed by the NOVA organization) is posted outside the dining room door. It's useful to know what to expect at meals so we can plan our day. Each day we must cross the street several times to get to the dining room. We are forced by the physical surroundings (not by someone's order or by rules) to be alert and moving. Such naturally occurring boundaries and stimuli are important adjuncts to therapy.

At dinner (chicken, coleslaw, peach cobbler, corn, and a biscuit) I began to consider the behavioral consequences of various serving styles. At B Home, for example, the serving style rewards those who rush in to get the prime seats, where one is served first. Also at B Home one's table mates pass the plates along to the far end of the table in a cooperative effort. Since here the food is already at one's place when one enters the dining room, the rush is avoided but so is the cooperative symbolism.

This evening, as I think over the research that has been done on these settings, I decide that much, if not all, of it may be based on a serious mistake. Facilities are usually classified by the number of residents. For example, family-care units have six or fewer residents; larger facilities are designated as board-and-care homes, halfway houses, and the like. But it is not the size of the facility which is the critical element in predicting the patient's success in adapting to the community. Rather, the style of the setting is the important feature, for some family-care units are as impersonal and businesslike as board-and-care homes. Conversely, a large board-and-care home may have enough informal subgroup systems to make life almost homey for its residents. Therefore, future comparative studies should look not only at structural features, such as size, in classifying aftercare facilities, but also at functional and expressive aspects.

Sunday, December 3

One of my roommates is beginning to deteriorate. I overheard him telling a friend that he had run out of medicine several days ago. I greeted him on the stairs but got no reply. My self-reflective response is to consider what condition I'd be in without Elavil.

There were only five or six others eating breakfast at 7 o'clock this morning. I really won't know how many residents are here until we have a popular meal on a weekday evening.

Several residents stood and saluted the flag in the corner of the lounge when our national anthem was played during the opening ceremony of the football game on TV. A couple of us didn't think it necessary and remained seated. A couple of others stopped midway through the ceremony and sat down. We had participated in the miscarriage of a mini custom.

M. is a sort of leader in the lounge. He makes his opinions and desires known to all. Today he yelled at people leaving or entering the room to leave the door open because it was hot inside. There was only one mild dissent, but the fellow who had spoken up quickly backed down ("I was only kidding") and the door stayed open.

F. came in and chewed out a resident for leaving his car in the driveway. It was the third time he had done so. She threatened to have the car towed away next time. She seemed unusually upset and slightly brittle as she shouted at him, almost out of control. I was mildly stunned.

There were sixteen men eating soup and bologna sandwiches for lunch. Those who arrived later than noon must inevitably get cold soup, since it is served all at once.

This afternoon I went for a walk into town. S Manor is ideally located in a residential section near snack shops, bowling alleys, theaters, and stores. Moreover, it is only fifteen to twenty minutes' walk away from a major shopping area with a mall and a beach. Getting away from the residence and losing oneself in the anonymity of the pedestrian role is a welcome change of pace. The size of the area that is within walking distance might surprise the automobile-addicted Californian.

Monday, December 4

I hurried to breakfast at 6:45, but the cook didn't open the dining hall until shortly after 7 o'clock. It was raining. I shared my umbrella with the resident who was to guide me to the bus stop. He usually catches the 7:06 A.M. municipal bus to the VA, sometimes even missing breakfast to do so. We were resigned to missing the early bus and catching the next one, but the bus was late, pulling up just as we got to the bus stop. My new friend was very solicitous. He offered all the necessary information about bus numbers, stops, and routes. He was worried that I wouldn't be able to get back home on my own. I reassured him, however, and we parted in the rain at the VA.

I returned to the manor from the VA just in time for dinner. As I rushed over to the dining hall, another resident was rushing, too. He asked what time it was. I told him it was 5:25. He said, "She likes to close about this time." But, I thought, the information sheet says we have until 5:30 P.M. to get in for dinner. The dining hall was open. I ate hurriedly but the other fellow took his time, even going back for seconds.

I went directly to the TV room to watch the Monday night football game. About seven or eight others were settling down to watch. I'm impressed by the intense patriotism of many veteran mental patients; they display a kind of "American Legionism." Lou Rawls, a black singer, sang the national anthem in a modern style, which some residents felt was "disgraceful." A large part of a patient's positive self-image seems to be tied to his seeing himself as a war hero of a great nation.

Tuesday, December 5

After breakfast I sat in the dining hall for a few minutes, deep in thought. To be honest, I'm having trouble making my depression look real in this facility. It may be that I've gotten away from the setting too frequently (both spatially and through books and television). It may be that a sense of familiarity with this neighborhood recalls my other identity. It may be that I've become satiated with depression or that I fear and resist its coming again. At any rate, I feel alone here, and yet I don't particularly mind the loneliness, as I usually do when I'm depressed. Nevertheless, there are irritations. When I entered I was promised that a pole would be put in my closet, but it has not yet been done. Nor have I received my ninety-five cents in change. The managers don't care.

I sat in the patio reading. JD, the male manager, came and went but did not greet me. The foreign cook and a handyman passed by, but they also ignored me. What a chilly social world!

The big red setter came up to me. As I started to reach out to pet him, someone called in a sharp voice, "Rex! Come here!" The dog obediently ran into the house. The door closed.

Later I went to the door. I said, "I think you owe me ninety-five cents." "I'll have to check and give it to you tomorrow, Okay?" F. replied after a pause. I was dismissed. As I turned away she closed the door in a way that seemed symbolic of her desire to close me out of her existence so I wouldn't bother her.

My roommate told me that there was a pool table in the room over the dining hall. I went there but couldn't get in because both the front and back doors were locked. I knocked on the kitchen door. The cook confirmed the existence of the pool table but said the room was kept locked. She spoke sympathetically, however, and used my name twice. I felt so good about talking with her that I paid scant attention to the negative content of what she said.

I sat outside in the patio reading. My disturbed roommate came and sat in the chair next to mine (though he could have selected another chair some distance away). We didn't talk at all but simply sat together. A fellow came to pick up his mail, but there wasn't any for him. He rang the bell to the manager's house and waited. How formal and distant and demeaning is this procedure! Ring the bell and wait to be recognized and handled.

During the mid-afternoon coffee break the cook was chatting with several of us in her Southern down-to-earth style. One resident used to drink heavily with the result that three years ago, when he came here after being released from the hospital, his social worker instructed the management to give him only ten dollars a week as spending money from his own funds. He hasn't touched a drink in two years and is completely unable to drink now because of an inner ear equilibrium problem, but still he can't get the extra five dollars a week he wants for spending. "Ask; you'll never get it if you don't ask for it," someone told him. That's a significant statement about having one's needs met in this setting. The cook advised him to see his social worker.

The cook joked about putting out a cup into which we could drop coins for her for Christmas, ending with "and no pennies, either." She told one fellow she'd let him off easy — he need only get her a sweater costing six dollars at Penney's. They joked about the cheap bulk Christmas presents they get each year from the wealthy owner of this residence. He drives both a Cadillac and a Lincoln Continental. I doubt that anyone even considers giving the owner a present.

The cook pointed out that the former alcoholic still isn't eating well. He told us he had lost weight and that he was now down to 139 pounds. This group reveals genuine mutual concern for one another.

T., my disturbed roommate, came in about 2:15 P.M. "You're late, T.," the cook said, "but we'll let it slide this time." She smiled. T. smiled.

Wednesday, December 6

I went to my "detail" at the VA and stayed until noon. After lunch I passed the young managers in the street; they ignored me. I sat in their yard twice. I know they were there because the phone rang and someone answered it. But no one called me in to give me the ninety-five cents they still owe me. This young couple may be going through some crisis of health or family conflict. They are strongly self-focused, and they seem unwilling to open up their world to others.

I walked by the lounge and suddenly realized that the ancient rerun movies these fifty- and sixty-year-old residents were watching are the movies of their youth. The movies and their stars have a special meaning for elderly residents which I can't share.

My roommate is friendly and informative, but his information is inexact. For example, what he told me about the pool table and the laundry is inaccurate. In life as well as in anthropology one must pick informants with care and check their replies against those of others.

At 1:45 P.M. I went for coffee. I walked into the dining room and noticed that no other resident was there. "Oh, I guess I'm early." The cook smiled and said that it was all right. She invited me to sit down and have a cup of coffee. Her orientation is toward people, not rules. We talked together for ten or fifteen minutes before the other residents arrived. She told me her life story. She had worked in restaurants and hospitals since she was fourteen. The last place was a convalescent home. One day when she was feeding oatmeal to an old lady the manager came over and started shoving huge spoonfuls into the lady's mouth to hurry her up. The cook walked back to the kitchen and out the door and never went back.

A former resident came in and got coffee. Some residents help the cook with dishes and buy her Cokes. She's a simple, charming lady who has had a rough life involving drinking and a broken marriage. But she is warm and kind and motherly.

Five or six fellows from my ward were waiting for the nurses to come for group therapy that afternoon. They were eager for the activity. Several were dressed up, some had stayed off their jobs, and all seemed enthusiastic about this weekly break in the routine. A number of places were considered as possible meeting sites: an upstairs room, the yard, a nearby hot dog stand. They waited anxiously. Finally, one ventured, "They're not coming." Another replied, "No, there's still time." As they waited one man expressed his belief that he couldn't have a wife because he feels he is not yet responsible enough. Later he clarified his position on marriage. He couldn't get married now — "Not while I'm nuts." Several were discussing the advantages and disadvantages of marriage, their unhappy experiences with women, and so forth. They were already creating the atmosphere of self-revelation, interested listening, and mental health topics — all requisite for a good group therapy meeting — when the nurses finally arrived, late.

One guy wandered around pitifully from person to person pleading for fifty cents, then a quarter, but he was turned down over and over again.

Thursday, December 7

I ate breakfast, took no medication, and left. I returned at 9:45 that night. No one mentioned my being gone at lunch and supper. No one mentioned my missing both morning and afternoon medications.

I had lost my key sometime that evening. Luckily, the door to our room was unlocked. T. was in bed asleep. My other roommate (I still don't know his name) was out somewhere. The wastebaskets were empty.

Friday, December 8

T. said I could get another key from the manager; he always does that when he loses his key. But I wanted to have it duplicated myself.

After duplicating my roommate's key I felt very relieved. When I assume my depressed identity unintended failures seriously upset me. They are signals that the depression and the identity are real and therefore are not completely under David Reynolds's control.

As I turned in my dishes after lunch the cook said, "Hello, David. How are you?" She smiled. "Okay," I said as I shuffled out. She cares.

I rang the bell of the managers' house. F. answered the door. "Do you have the ninety-five cents?" I asked. She didn't say a word, left me standing on the doorstep, and closed the door in my face as she went to get the money. She gave it to me. I said, "Also, there's still no pole in my closet. Also, next Thursday I'm going to live with my friend." "All right," she said, showing no interest. She closed the door. I felt her coldness and rigidity. Her reaction to me might have stemmed from her fear of the difference she perceived between us.

I began to think about what kind of cues I would get if people became aware of my alternate identity, showing that my cover had been broken. Certainly, if the managers here had been aware of the research I was doing they would have installed my closet pole and would promptly have given me the change they owed me. Why? Because they would perceive that I have more power than most residents and would treat me accordingly. Too bad!

At 2 P.M. I went to the coffee break. The cook asked me, "You didn't eat here last night, did you, David?" She had noticed my absence. How pleased I felt! I told her I had been to my friend's apartment and would probably move soon. She was interested in my leaving. My "together" roommate has been gone a lot lately. He isn't watching TV as usual; he comes in late at night and leaves soon after breakfast. I wonder if my announcement that I won't be staying here very long has anything to do with the change in him. I asked T., the other fellow, about his being gone. Because our roommate is sleeping here at night, T. is not worried about him; he even seems unconcerned.

I left S Manor after supper and didn't return until breakfast the next day. Nobody mentioned my absence.

Saturday, December 9

Tonight there was the usual chatter at supper and the predictable line of chairs in front of the TV in the lounge. One resident decided to go to a movie. Another volunteered to walk with him but then decided to see a different film. A resident carried out the overflowing trash can from the lounge. That's how it was, and that's how it would continue to be, evening after evening. I left.

Walking to my car I realized the uniqueness of this experience, of walking around knowing I'm different from other people. It is more than recognizing that other people see me as different. I *am* different. The fact that I exist with this life style in this sheltered, simplified preserve is both evidence for and a symbol of that difference. I pay for society's handout with loss of self-esteem and belongingness. That recognition is wearing and tiresome. And when I can't escape from it any longer with sleep or television or immersion in the little aftercare society that feigns normalcy, I sometimes feel like adopting a permanent solution, the irreversible one. Or I toy with the idea of taking enough pills to hurt but not kill myself because then, for a while at least, I'll be a truly sick human and not a crazy one.

I returned to my room at 9:45 P.M. and turned off the portable radio that had been playing since 6 o'clock that evening; my roommate, T., had been asleep all the time.

Sunday, December 10

I got two butter patties at breakfast when I was handed my pancakes. Strange how important that seemed. I looked around to see if I had been singularly privileged. Does this cook like me, too? I ignored my medication. Told my "together" roommate I hadn't seen him around much lately. He said he's been out a lot, ". . . visiting, you know."

It is 9 A.M. and I sit here writing notes. T. is in the rocking chair this morning, chuckling over some internal, unshareable event. The other guy is asleep. Sometimes T. shakes his head back and forth when he thinks no one is looking. Freedom to respond impulsively to inner urges is a privilege of mental disorder, and one might as well cash in on it since one pays the price for it, hour by hour. T. gets up and leaves, returning ten minutes later. The other guy lies in bed passing huge bursts of intestinal gas.

T. has brought back a quart of wine. He offers me some and we sit, drinking and talking. He has been here since last April or May. I don't know how much of the rest of his conversation is objectively true. He said that he had been a lieutenant in the navy, that he had six cars last year (naming them), that he sued Buick for $200,000, and that he will draw service pay until his retirement sometime in the future. He drank most of the bottle of wine, then went into the bathroom and vomited up every drop.

On the way to morning coffee break, several of us crossed the street in the middle of the block in front of a police car. Who cares if we get a ticket for jaywalking? What can they do to us? But we all hurried into the dining hall when we saw the car pull up to the curb farther up the block.

Monday, December 11

Shortly after lunch the managers knocked on the door. "We've got to inspect your room," F. said as she led the way in. "Good-morning," J. said. I sat down again. They went into the bathroom, staying for only a few seconds, and then left. Perhaps they were checking the toilet; it's been leaking on the floor for a week.

I took a long walk down by the pier and shipping area. David Randolph has a very self-indulgent attitude toward life. I find myself growing lax in self-discipline, as manifested in my unwillingness to write notes or to resist buying things. The compulsive productivity of my other self seems very far away.

Tuesday, December 12

The medicine cups from breakfast remain by the coffee urn so that if we forgot before, we can take the pills at lunch. Interestingly, taking or not taking medication has become a symbolic gesture of personal control over my life. Sometimes I don't take the pills just because I don't have to.

That evening, passing T. in the street, I asked, "How's dinner?" I got no reply. T. simply ignored me.

Wednesday, December 13

After breakfast I wandered into the lounge. Two resident leaders were planning what R. would say to the managers about residents' requests for a Christmas party. R. took a rather conservative position, whereas the other man aimed at getting all we could out of the owner.

The topics discussed covered a wide field. (1) "Young girls," not "bags," should be invited to the party. (2) Residents should dress presentably. (3) Attendance should not be mandatory. (4) There should be presents for everybody, and they should not be cheap. (5) Residents should volunteer to assist in putting up decorations in the lounge so as not to overburden the managers. (6) There should be a real Christmas tree in the lounge. (7) There should be special lighting for the party. (8) The managers should be there to help.

Discussion shifted to an evaluation of the managers. "I like 'em all right, but I've never seen 'em come in here," R. said (meaning that the managers do not participate in the residents' activities). One of the managers had been working at another of the owner's facilities from noon until 4 P.M., he thought, but someone said she had quit there. There was a consensus that the managers and owner are "slippery" characters and will finagle themselves out of responsibilities whenever they can get away with it. R. noted that the owner claims he's going broke. Everybody laughed. "With that crooked bookkeeper of his I don't see how he can," somebody said. The residents decided not to approach the managers yet. It was 8:30 A.M. "They're not up now; no use getting them mad."

The ex-boxer is afraid to go back to the hospital. He hasn't slept in two nights and worries that the hospital authorities will keep him there when they find out about his insomnia. A few days earlier he got into a fight with another resident. The other fighter's lip was cut, and he called the police. The ex-boxer hadn't seemed particularly upset at the time. He had been in trouble before and he would be in trouble again, he figured. But now he hesitated to go back to the hospital for his regular checkup.

From noon until 1:30 P.M. the lounge door was locked while the managers decorated. When the door opened we gazed at a small artificial tree, a few strands of glittering rope, and a plastic Merry Christmas sign.

M. didn't plan on coming to the Christmas party because it starts at 8 P.M., and that's his bedtime. The cook vowed to get him up this time, though. He said he wouldn't get up, but she kidded him that he must get up in order to put his present for her under the tree.

At 5 P.M. the dinner seemed hurried. The cooks, even our lovable Southerner, bustled around in uncommunicative fashion, wiping off the tables as soon as people had finished eating.

I read and slept. Tomorrow will be my third day without a shower.

Thursday, December 14

I don't mind leaving here today. Am I used to separations now? Is it because I'll be away from the managers? Two weeks were long enough to establish a sense of belongingness and a feeling of being wrenched away when I left the psychiatric ward. This time it is different.

After lunch I told the cook I was leaving tonight. "Where are you going?" she asked. "Will you move in with your friend?" "Yes," I said. "Where's that, in Santa Monica or Los Angeles?" she asked. I replied that it's in West Los Angeles. She said she was sorry to see me go.

I rang the managers' bell. F. came to the door and stood in the doorway. I asked, "Do I have any mail?" "No," she replied. "I'm going to leave after dinner tonight," I said. "Okay, fine," she said with an unconcerned air. "Will you be here so I can give you the key?" I asked. "Yes, I'll be here," she replied. "Okay," I said. I turned away. F. makes me very angry. Her hardness, her disinterest, her lack of compassion, and her lack of minimal social grace, combined with her power over the residents' lives, are upsetting to me. She could be doing a great deal for them and for herself, but she's not.

I told T. that I'm leaving tonight, but there was no response.

I sat in the yard reading. F. came out and yelled for the dog. The setter didn't come immediately, ignoring the woman's calls which became louder and louder until she was practically screaming. She has no patience when things don't go her way.

At the afternoon coffee break the Greek cook (who is also the maid) asked me when I was leaving so she could change my bed. I learned that the number of residents has declined recently. The cook complained that her meat order had been cut back and she would have to start putting filler in it, as they do at the owner's other places.

F. breezed in to tack up a Christmas party poster. "Speak English!" she said, half annoyed, half joking, to the Greek cook and the resident who were talking in their native language. F. ignored us, went about her business, and left.

At 2:20 P.M. I met T. outside on the sidewalk. He said he was going to go to UCLA, that he had played football for UCLA last spring. He said there was to be a party on Saturday, but he had the day wrong. I told him and another fellow that I would be leaving tonight. "But I'll come back and visit sometime." Without replying they turned and walked away in different directions.

There were four farewells that evening. As I turned in my supper dishes the cook said, "Take care now." I told her good-bye.

I returned to my room for my suitcase. T. was sitting in the rocking chair listening to his radio. "I'm leaving, now, T. Bye," I said. He mumbled something. I stopped. He repeated the mumble. "What?" I asked. He gave up the attempt at talking and just nodded and smiled. It was the best he could do at the moment. I smiled, too, and said, "Bye, T."

I took my key to the managers' house and told F. I was leaving. Then I had to remind her of my medication. She said, "Oh, yes," and went back to get it. I asked if I could come back for the Christmas party on Sunday evening. It was a hard thing for me to do, because I feared another rejection. But she replied, "Yes! By all means! Come back anytime."

Passing by the TV lounge I put my head in the door. Half a dozen residents were watching television and talking. I called in softly, "Bye now." One fellow called back, "Have a nice Christmas. Shut the door, will ya?" It was a fitting end to my stay at S Manor.

Postscript: A Christmas Party

The party was scheduled for 8 o'clock on a Sunday evening. I arrived at 7:45. Nearly twenty residents had gathered in the TV lounge. No attempt had been made to rearrange the chairs, which were lined up as usual in front of the TV set. Someone had brought in a radio to provide music for the evening.

There was nervous, sometimes vulgar, conversation about women as the men nervously awaited their encounter with the opposite sex. It was the jittery atmosphere that one finds among freshman hopefuls before a high school dance. Several guys wanted to watch the Walt Disney program on television until 8 o'clock, but M. wouldn't allow it: "They'll think we're a bunch of fags."

A few minutes after 8 the door by the TV opened and F. and her girl friend appeared. F. announced that the NOVA organizer had been unable to get UCLA girls to come to the party. So on Friday she had invited women from a board-and-care home. They had accepted the invitation but called later to decline. Dr. W. might bring some girls. But F. had contacted two other girl friends who would arrive shortly.

F. passed out Christmas presents (shaving lotion, as is customary here). I was somewhat surprised to get a gift, too. As she passed out the presents, she checked the names off a list.

After a few minutes in which we just sat, F. announced that punch and hors d'oeuvres were in the next room. Silently we filed in to get the refreshments. In that room sat F.'s husband, J., a VA employee who used to work at S Manor, and a young couple.

I took my food back to a chair in the lounge. T. passed by, smiled, and pressed my shoulder. The radio was playing. I talked with F.'s friend for a few minutes.

By 8:30 F.'s other friends had arrived. They soon picked up the style of interaction which restricted their attention to the two managers, the young couple, and the other ladies. After each of the three lady guests had danced once or twice with a resident (and only two or three residents were bold enough to ask, having seen others turned down), they grouped themselves together for in-group conversation.

By 9:15 only nine residents were still at the party. Half an hour later the three ladies were talking together, seated in a circle at the center of the TV lounge; the nine residents were ranged around the wall. The radio was playing — mockingly. By 10:15 the segregation was complete, with all the residents in the lounge and all the "normals" in the next room. One fellow had brought out a bowl of mixed chips and was solemnly picking through them for his favorite cheese nibbles.

F. announced that we had only twenty minutes to finish eating; then she was going to take the leftovers home. She was talking with her friends about some of the case histories of the residents. One lady told her we had run out of punch. "I don't want to make any more," F. replied. "Anyway, how can you drink that stuff?"

I talked with the residents. Last year's party was much more successful, it seems. "I feel like I've been turned down at a 'dime-a-dance,' " one young fellow mourned wryly. It was a flop, "a big flop" another one felt.

At 10:20 there were eight residents and eight of the others left, still segregated neatly in separate rooms. I left. Someone had stolen my present.

S MANOR DEBRIEFING

NLF: Let me tell you what this meeting is about. About six or eight months ago, you may recall, at a meeting held at the hospital it was announced that research was being conducted to discover what happened to mental patients after their release from the hospital, and that managers of aftercare facilities who wanted to participate in the program could sign up as sponsors. The study would begin sometime within the next six months or so. We would then tell you about it, see what your impressions were, keep you informed about the kinds of things we were interested in, and get your reactions. I would like to ask you, then, whether or not you can identify any resident placed in this way in S Manor within the past six to eight months as a patient who was recently released from the hospital.

FD: Discharged from the hospital, you mean?

NLF: He had been in the hospital and had been discharged.

FD: No, I can't think of anybody that has been discharged.

JD: Can you picture anyone we've had in the past six months who may have been placed here as a patient but who was not a patient? Who was here just to observe?

FD: Oh . . .

JD: . . . and I can only say that I have no suspicion.

NLF: That's very good.

FD: No, because we've had only about three placements in the past six months, if that many.

NLF: I see. That should make it easier for you.

FD: We've had a couple of the undercover guys?

NLF: Yes, it sounds like undercover stuff, and that puts a little tinge of excitement into it, but the whole basis for it was our deep interest in suicidal patients. Especially we want to discover what happens to people who have been suicidal and were treated in the hospital and then were released. While they were in the hospital, they seemed to be able to handle themselves pretty well; but often when they are released from the hospital, they seem to run into problems, and then they find themselves in positions of stress and difficulties which they haven't been able to take in stride. Then they begin to lose their control and their ability to adjust. We have been trying to — we talk with a lot of these people and get their impressions and get information from them about what happens. But we also felt that it would be very helpful to have somebody who is not a mental patient go through the same experience. For that task we have a trained person — trained as an anthropologist. Anthropologists often go out into the field, usually to study a tribe or a foreign place, especially a very primitive place, and live with the people and learn how the people get along together. It's also true that anthropologists go to subcommunities in various places in an effort to get a personal feeling and understanding of the kind of culture and subculture those people experience. If I may, I would like to ask our anthropologist and his social worker to come in.

FD: Oh, for God's sake! You! You!

NLF: This man is David Reynolds.

FD: Dianna [one of her girl friends] said, "He's so intelligent!"

JD: Well, I heard him talk in Japanese.

FD: Undercover man! Would you like a cup of coffee?

NLF: I started to tell Mr. and Mrs. D. about the experiential research. We have carried out this research in several places in order to get the personal reaction of a thoroughly trained person who knows what to look for and who can also look at himself and see what's happening to his own feelings as he goes through these experiences. It's very interesting, then, that neither of you had any kind of reaction to David, especially. . . Tell me how you saw him. What were your feelings about him?

JD: He was mostly quiet. I learned most about him at the Christmas party, I think.

DKR: Yes, that's right. I allowed myself to be my other self a little more at the Christmas party.

FD: And my girl friend, I know, talked to him for a while. She said, "He is so intelligent!" And then she asked, "What's he doing in a place like this?"

KF: [social worker]: Now you can tell her.

FD: Sneaky, sneaky, sneaky.

KF: I thought maybe you would have remembered that he was in our ward a year ago. Same thing; he came as a patient as part of a study.

NLF: As part of the study we also included experience in the hospital, so David spent some time actually as a suicidal patient in the ward without anybody knowing who he really was.

JD: I think I heard that was coming up but I don't remember.

FD: I remember . . .

DKR: The experiment is really more than just role playing or faking. I become genuinely depressed and make myself suicidal, and so I'm not just acting.

FD: I know. Being around them [mental patients], after a while, especially at this time of year, everybody gets depressed. They come and say "Oh, I haven't any Christmas cards, I haven't heard from my family," and they just sit there.

NLF: Do you have any other depressed or suicidal people at S Manor at present?

FD: I don't believe we have.

JD: There's one that we have to keep an eye on — that's R.

FD: He's the only one that's suicidal, but we haven't had any problems with him. It's been more than a year and we've only had two [suicide] attempts, one major and one minor.

FD: Do any of the fellows know about you? They don't know about you, do they?

DKR: Those are some of the things we would like to ask you. We'd like to know your perspective on whether or not we ought to tell them.

FD: I don't think it's necessary. They might not like it.

JD: Well, they are all highly suspicious anyway. G. never forgets anything. I don't think it's necessary.

DKR: I thought I might tell you something about my experiences. And we'd like you to tell us how you saw the situation, so that we can get different perspectives on the same situation. That's part of the reason we are here, because we know that one person's view of anything is distorted and we need your perspective. The most pleasant and warmest experiences I had while I was at S Manor were at the very beginning and the very end of my stay. When I first came, your orientation procedures were very good. When a person is a bit depressed, or when he is disturbed in some way, the information that people give him may not be filtering through very well. He's often very sensitive to feelings and attitudes in other people, but at the same time the comments aren't coming through to him. I think the written material that you provide is a useful kind of thing. I appreciated very much your introducing me to the resident who rides the bus to the VA. You introduced me as another person from his ward, and that immediately formed a bond and already started to get me into the little group of residents. It was a very warm feeling. Before I left, the last thing I did — I don't know if you remember — was to ask if I could come back to the Christmas party. I was afraid to ask that because I didn't think you liked me; I didn't think either of you liked me. But you said, "Yes, by all means, come back anytime." That produced warm feelings, too, and I left with a kind of glow. So those were the two exceptionally good points I would like to mention.

FD: I always tell everybody to come back because I know there are a lot of fellows who form a relationship, and when someone moves on and goes back to the hospital, I always tell them to come back. Why not? We're their friends and I'm sure most of these fellows are our friends.

DKR: I've been in several facilities now, and I think that generally speaking the facilities you have here, the furnishings, and the food are comparatively good. The cook is very open and friendly and she has good relationships with the residents. And she, like you, uses first names a lot. When somebody cares enough to learn my name and to call me by name — that's important.

There was discussion of medication, the 95 cents change owing David Randolph, and the promised pole that was never installed in his closet.

NLF: Some of your people become long-term residents.

FD: They make it permanent. We have, I would say, at least six or eight who could go out and get their own apartments and live on their own with no trouble at all, not even financial trouble, but they choose to stay here. I guess they like the protected environment.

NLF: Yes, I guess they're able to make friends and are able to stay with friends in this way.

JD: Like J. The cleaning woman does his laundry. He gets his meals. He doesn't even want to get well. He's quite content to watch TV all day.

NLF: Is there any pressure for them to move out in any way?

JD: Yes, the state, I think, puts more pressure on them than the VA because the state-sponsored welfare program sends medical fliers to make them prove they're still completely disabled.

DKR: On the next point, I very much need your perspective. I sensed a kind of distance and coolness during most of my stay in S Manor. It was almost as if you seemed distracted. After leaving I learned that part of the philosophy of S Manor is to make the residents as independent as possible. You're supposed to keep this kind of distance so that they don't become overdependent on you. The way that distance affected me, though — it hit me as if you really didn't care much about me. I would have preferred friendliness, even of a distant kind.

FD: You wanted us to be more talkative?

DKR: Well, at least gestures like a friendly greeting on the street, using my name as you did, the orientation you had, introducing other residents — that sort of thing. I didn't care about long discussions because I could have come here at any time. But those vague signals of friendliness. Let me give you an example of how that affected me. One day I was out sitting in the chair and your dog was out there. I started to reach out to pet him, and just when I started you called, "Rex," and you opened the door and Rex ran in. I know it must have been the time for the dog to eat or you wanted Rex in the house for some other reason; but I was getting paranoid that nobody really cared about me and I didn't have any contact with you, just business matters, and I thought, "Oh, my gosh, you don't want me bothering Rex," and I felt very sad about that.

JD: Well, that's another area. Rex, out there in the yard. Now he's a nervous wreck, he's outgoing, he'll run you ragged, and there are a few of the fellows like M. He really likes Rex but he's afraid of him, not sure of him, so it's kind of putting him on someone, and, like I say, your stay here was so short that we didn't really get to know you. And that's usually what we do. I still say "Good-morning" to E. whenever I pass him and I don't think he's ever replied. That I would do, you know. And I figure one day he's going to say "Hi" back, and I'll probably fall over. A lot of them are very standoffish, and it seems to be imposing on their privacy to say just "Hello" to them.

NLF: I think what David may be talking about in terms of his feelings is the difference between being standoffish and, I guess, being formal and proper and so on and being withdrawn in a psychological sense. You can be withdrawn because you are afraid or because you are paranoid and you feel that people don't like you, and you always have your antenna up and so on, so that the first person, the very proper person, would resent any kind of greetings and friendliness. But the second person would be very concerned and very sensitive about not getting any, and the difficulty occurs in terms of being able to sense that difference.

JD: T. is very much like that. In one sense, he would never initiate a greeting, but I'm sure he appreciates greetings from others.

NLF: Yes, that's it exactly.

FD: When was it — last year, last Christmas, and before and after — we had all those young guys here and they would come and they'd want to talk. Well, J. and I would talk to them. Or at times when J. wasn't here, I would talk to them. Anyway, there were several of them that never really got out of line with me. They were very friendly. A few of them said, "It's too bad that you're married, but I wouldn't ask you out or anything because of J. and I appreciate J." There was one fellow that I didn't get involved with but I felt sorry for him and I would listen to him. And he got too attached to me. I finally had to turn away from him. So since then I kind of have my guard up. I don't want to spend a lot of time because I can't take it, to be very honest with you. You know, they start telling me about their past sex problems and their girl friends, and I'm sitting there and — Oh, God, what am I going to do? When I don't know somebody, I try to keep my guard up. Now I've learned, you know. I am careful because I can't take it. I end up crying and blubbering so I keep my distance now. With J., you know, it's different; he can talk to them, which he did several times with this one fellow. I don't get close to the residents as I used to. I try to be friendly and make them feel at home, and, of course, if they need anything, I tell them to please come and see us. I don't care what time it is, but I don't want to — I keep a distance. It is sad.

DKR: There are many people who don't need the intimate signals, but when they're depressed they need the little signals that say they're worth something, that somebody else thinks they're worth something. Because that's part of the problem they're facing. They're debating whether they are worth keeping alive or not, and it's other people who help them decide.

FD: Well, it also depends on the person because I used to have a bad habit of saying, "Hi, how are you? Everything okay?" Dr. W. explained to me about the touching. One person would take it as friendship and the next person would think, hmmm, she touched me, so I broke away from that. When I like somebody I also say, "Hi, how are you, everything okay?" — just friendship. To me, it's friendly. But they can turn it around, especially if they start to go downhill. So I watch, which I don't like. I like to be friendly and let them know I care.

NLF: It's a difficult line to follow without getting overinvolved and yet without being overdetached.

KF: I'd rather have my job than your job because there's no separation, twenty-four hours a day. I have an automatic time schedule that allows me to keep some distance, but you don't.

FD: We're here all the time, you know.

NLF: Residents, too, stay a long, long time and you become "family." You can't help it.

FD: No, I give them hell just as a mother does. You know, J. gets mad at me and says to leave them alone, you're not their mother, but I can't help it. It's motherly instinct, I think, in a woman, to be warm and kind of protective even though in the long run it doesn't work; so I watch now. I try not to be like that and it's hard. 'Cause there are a lot of them here to whom, especially at this time of year, I want to say, "Oh, gee, come on home with me," or whatever, but you can't.

DKR: I'm struck by the difficulty of this kind of work and also the importance of your role in the lives of the residents. You know, I was part of their world, and I know that they were important to me, too. But somehow a lot of mental patients have the same stereotypes as other people do about mental illness and the same idea of stigma associated with it. So when "normal" people seem to care about you, there's something extra about that. It's a very hard tightrope to walk.

FD: Oh, it is, because you don't want to get involved, yet you do. You're back and forth. It's hard. That's why I was standoffish.

DKR: That's really all the information that I'd like to pass along to you. Is there anything else you can recall about your interactions with me that would help us to understand whether I did seem to you to be really depressed or whether I didn't?

FD: Well, now, J. would notice that. I wouldn't. I don't know if the residents are depressed. I know if they're getting withdrawn a little bit and a little depressed. But with you, I thought you were just quiet and a loner. That was my impression. I never thought of you as being suicidal. I thought you preferred to be alone. I didn't really want to intrude.

NLF: Suppose he had made a suicidal attempt, what would have been your procedure? What would you have done?

JD: It depends on the kind of attempt.

NLF: Yes, of course. Well, let's say that it didn't require any medical attention.

JD: We would call KF . . . and get a team out here for that. We don't have an emergency team, you know. We haven't got any troubleshooting facility whatsoever with the exception of the police department; that is our only recourse, and then the resident would have to break a law before we can call the police. So if we have somebody that is acting strangely and is not hurting anyone, whether he's threatening to or not, we don't have any recourse but to wait until he does something. I think that's a hell of a gap that the VA should fill. They should have some kind of troubleshooting team out of admissions or somewhere.

FD: We used at least to have the nurses out. We don't have them anymore.

JD: I know if we call the nurses out, they can't transport the patients or anything so there's nothing we can do until a patient hits someone, breaks something, or . . .

KF: You might tell them about what you've done with your uncle. It's a good example of how you worked out that problem.

JD: Well, I have an uncle on the police force. I have called him on occasion, and he'll send someone out and usually, in almost 90 percent of the cases, the minute the patients see the uniform and recognize authority, they'll settle down and will go to the hospital either with me or with the unit. It's not official because they haven't broken a law.

NLF: Do you have recourse in terms of getting them back into the hospital if they are suicidal?

JD: If a patient refuses to go to the hospital, I can't do anything. I can call the social worker, and he'll come out and maybe he can talk the patient into going back. K., being a male, has an advantage; a male social worker has a little more authority than a female in trying to get a patient back to the hospital.

FD: We had a fellow here, Mr. G., who got to the point where he wouldn't eat. He'd walk around, but he just wouldn't eat and he kept losing weight and was skinny to begin with. Miss J. came out. She happened to come out that day. Between us she and I spent almost an hour and a half trying to get somebody from the hospital, anywhere, to come and take and move this fellow. Now, he wasn't being hostile; he wasn't withdrawn. I mean he did talk if you spoke to him. And he would walk around. He would walk back and forth. But he just wasn't eating, and he got to the point where we were afraid if he did fall, he would break every bone in his body. It was about an hour and a half we spent on the phone. Miss J. talked to admissions, and we talked to the police department. We finally got hold of the mental health clinic. She was on the phone, I don't know how long, with them. She told them who she was, what the fellow's name was, and gave them all the information. They finally came up, but they don't even have the pickup service now. You have to take patients in yourself. And the last two times the police department was out to help us, they wouldn't take the patient to the VA. They took him down to the mental health clinic.

JD: Well, I can see why, because if they take him to admissions, they have to sit there for an hour or so and that's taking them out of service. They really don't think it's their job. I tend to agree with them.

FD: But it's quite frustrating when you see someone going down the tubes and not getting help. Now you'll come out, you know, if you have any troubles with fellows from your ward. You're trying to do something about it, but there's nothing you can do until they go all the way.

JD: We had lots of support from the hospital before from that sponsors' program when everybody was supposed to get more and more help because expenses were going down at the hospital. But it's less and less now. Dr. W. used to come here once a week. He was very helpful, but that program was stopped.

FD: Dr. G. tried to get us involved in one of his programs.

JD: But it was the other way around — we had to go to the hospital two or three times a week.

DKR: So you feel that as time goes on there is less and less support for you right here.

JD: The hospital takes the patients up to discharge and then after discharge they don't get any help.

FD: As an example, consider RM, who was suicidal. They told us, I don't know how many times, the minute he stops taking his medication, phone his social worker, phone the nurse, and let the doctor know. So we did. So, in the past, all these people would come out and talk to R. He's been out of medication now for about a month. I phoned Mr. D. and he said, "I don't know what to tell you." So there you are — what do we do? We just wait till something happens. And he is highly suicidal, I gather from the nurses and the doctor. But the doctor says, "What can I do?" His hands are tied, too. I mean, he would come out and tell R., "Go to the hospital, go to the hospital, come out and get your medication." R. would go, but he would have to come out a few days in a row and give him the devil, but he would eventually go out to get his medication. Now, Mr. D. says, "I don't know what to tell you."

NLF: Why is that?

FD: I don't know.

KF: My only hunch is that they've had a lot of staff problems in that ward.

FD: When I phoned Mr. D. about M., I said, "He's been out of medication for about a month now." He said, "I don't know what to tell you." Any other time and he's out here like that.

NLF: Well, then, there are obviously a couple of ways in which more help could be given you. Can you think of any other things that you would find useful which you lack now?

FD: If we could just get somebody from the hospital to come out once a week or once every two weeks.

JD: I don't even know that it's necessary on a regular schedule, but if you just had someone we could phone to come down here to help.

NLF: Your concern would be to have some kind of facility for intervention before the person actually has done something drastic.

JD: Sure, it's so much easier for them to snap them back before they go all the way down.

FD: If you have to wait until they hit bottom, you know . . .

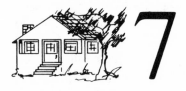

7 RECOMMENDATIONS TO SPONSORS

At the beginning of the project we agreed to present some of our findings to the aftercare sponsors' group that formed the pool from which we selected facilities for our live-in research. The findings, presented to the group in 1973, were published in the *California Association of Residential Care Homes News* in March 1975. This chapter presents an edited and enlarged version of our report to the sponsors. In it we focus on simple activities of everyday life in residential aftercare facilities and the special meanings those activities can have for a resident and the ways they can affect his life and his self-image.

Meals

Mealtime is an occasion that signifies more than eating. To the bored, inactive resident, food becomes a major part of his life. A surprisingly large portion of thinking and conversation in an aftercare facility centers on meals. The basic minimum obligation of owner or manager is to prepare good-tasting food and to serve it on time and under sanitary conditions. Some sponsors, however, wisely regarded mealtime as much more than an opportunity to feed residents. In some places the sponsors sought to ascertain their residents' food preferences so that diets could be planned accordingly. In this way they were communicating the information that individuals' tastes and choices were important. Some sponsors also showed concern by noticing lack of appetite (often a depressed person isn't hungry) or increases in appetite. The important thing was that sponsors who noticed such changes and commented on them were attentive to what was going on in the residents' world.

In one facility that was too large for the managers to heed individual habits of the residents, the cook alertly observed and commented on residents who failed to show up for meals. Another large facility had food-preference sheets. The managers did not have the time to talk with each resident individually, but they did ask the residents to fill out these sheets in order to communicate their wishes.

Some sponsors used mealtimes for getting people together and letting them talk. Sitting after a meal over a cup of coffee may be the only time that a resident can be assured of being around other people who are in a mood to talk. It is a social occasion in our society which allows people to converse in a comfortable atmosphere. The serving of meals makes a difference in the way that people relate, too. In some settings the purpose seems to be to get through the meal as quickly as possible, to herd people in and out fast. Family-style settings seemed most common. Self-service was often the rule and helped to hurry the pace. Posted regulations, which could be read to the new resident when he entered, helped to establish the amenities of a more social existence.

Sleeping Quarters

A room is more than a place to sleep. Many physical features of a room in a board-and-care home — closet space, drawer space, lighting, a comfortable mattress, a chair, a wastebasket, and so on — are important to a resident. But of more concern to the newcomer, particularly if he is depressed, are the social aspects of the room in which he is placed. The depressed person often tries to isolate himself from the rest of the world, and if he has a room where he can "hole up," where nobody is passing through and nobody else is around, he may sink into a deeper depression and thus cause even more concern than he otherwise would. It might therefore be wise to place a depressed person in a room where there will be some traffic and where other people will be present from time to time. In one of the facilities in which Kent lived, residents had to walk through a corner of his room to get to and leave another room. In other words, the traffic patterns of the rooms were used purposefully. State laws may now place limitations on such traffic patterns, but placement of withdrawn persons in rooms close to activities and staff is still possible.

The selection of a roommate for a suicidal resident should be carefully planned. Kent felt that some of his roommates were selected precisely because the sponsors thought they would be good companions for him. In the last place he stayed his roommate was a friendly, easygoing, talkative man who willingly gave information and advice and offered directions to Kent's desired destinations. Although the information was often wrong, the roommate served a larger purpose by providing concerned personal contact. The line between allowing a person privacy without meddling in his affairs and yet showing concern is a fine one. One of the ways to make sure that the resident gets needed contacts is careful selection of the room and the roommate.

Beds, Invitations, and Praise

Making beds is more than a simple housekeeping procedure; it can be used to establish rapport with a resident. The manager of one facility told Kent, "You don't have to make your bed here, but it will help if you do." She expected and encouraged him to be helpful in this way, but she didn't pressure him. Kent was also invited to answer the phone in that same facility, but he didn't have to do so. He was asked, "Tomorrow, if you feel like it, will you watch the phones for us?" And the next day, since he felt like it, he did. The encouragement, the opportunity, the invitation — all were there without the pressure.

In another place Kent was invited to go to church with the sponsor. At the same time he was permitted an honorable escape if he felt he wasn't up to making the effort. So he didn't have to feel like a failure. Depressed persons can find in almost everything they do, and in things they don't do, symbols of their hopelessness and worthlessness. Sometimes they even search for verification of their own uselessness.

Some of the facilities offered residents a lot of praise. A manager must be careful not to overpraise, for if people are praised for doing things that any child can do, they sense the artificiality. Kent was praised for doing things that deserved a response, such as carrying out worthwhile tasks. The taking on of responsibility is an option that should be offered to residents to help them grow.

Respect and Consideration

A resident deserves an explanation when the routine is disrupted or when he has been inconvenienced. He deserves to be treated with politeness, to be known by name, to be introduced to other people when he first enters, and to be helped in getting established in the residents' community.

In one family-care unit, good-natured joking supported the residents' sense of manhood. A resident got dressed up to go to church one morning. As he walked out the door, someone called to him, "Bring her back and let us see her," implying that he was actually going out to meet a woman. In a board-and-care home a resident complained to the cook, "Gee, I've given up with women." By responding, "You know, there might just be one right down the way for you," the cook was telling him that she saw him as a person with potential.

The resident is worthy of respect. He should be taken seriously until he proves that his word isn't dependable. In one facility the sponsor's car was giving her trouble — the engine made a pinging noise. One of the residents suggested that she use high-octane gas, saying that it might improve the performance of her car. She took him seriously, found that the idea was a good one, and thanked him for his help. The pool of experience-based knowledge in the corps of residents can be tapped if they are treated with respect and consideration.

In one home excellent advice was offered to a new assistant manager by an experienced sponsor. When the new employee complained that she was having problems with a certain resident, the sponsor advised, "You know, I think the best thing to do would be to sit down with him and have a cup of coffee and find out what's on his mind. If you listen carefully to what people are talking about, some problems just seem to evaporate."

Racial Problems

Two of the facilities in which Kent lived had black sponsors. In one facility Kent was the only white resident. At the first residence, after Kent had been there about half an hour, the sponsor said to him, "I know we're different colors, but among friends color doesn't matter, and I want to be your friend." She was a wise woman. She recognized that the difference in race might cause problems, but she deemed their personal relationship more important than the difference. In the other residence everyone pretended to ignore racial differences. As a result, feelings of discrimination and even mild paranoia, though never rising above the surface, caused unnecessary trouble. Facilities that accommodate members of different races would be well advised to bring the potential problem out into the open and deal with it straightforwardly.

Establishing Personal Relationships

Many staff members in mental hospitals and board-and-care homes emphasize the differences between themselves and the residents, whereas there are actually many similarities. The things shared with residents can help create a bond between staff and resident. For example, one sponsor spent the first couple of days and a major portion of their interaction in establishing the similarities between herself and Kent. She told him all sorts of ways in which they were alike, such as how she had gone through crises too and had needed help from other people. Those people had helped to pull her through her crises, and now that Kent was experiencing a crisis she was going to help him. It was okay, she said, to accept help. She also liked some of the same kinds of food that Kent liked; she held essentially the same religious beliefs as he did; and she also preferred to bathe before going to bed rather than showering in the morning. Over and over she emphasized the things they had in common. The message — "We are alike, I understand you, I'm concerned about you; I see you as another person" — came through clearly.

It is important to let the new resident know that the staff is experienced, that they know what they are doing, that they have expertise. Some staff members have certificates from sponsors' training programs; some have previously served as nurses; all of them have accumulated valuable experience in the daily carrying out of their duties. It is reassuring for the resident to know that the people with whom he is living are competent.

Staff members should be available to residents and should show interest in them and their problems. Two styles of management prevailed in the aftercare facilities in which Kent lived. One was a foster home whose manager or sponsor participated actively in the lives of the residents. She sought them out; she revealed her involvement in their lives; she took them with her when she went to the doctor or to church; she sought their company when she did her gardening or her cooking. The residents were with her almost all the time, a situation that was possible because the facility was fairly small.

The second management style was found in a larger place which was essentially a boardinghouse. The sponsors or managers were not active, but reactive. They waited in the office to consult with any resident who came by. A resident who had a problem was expected to come to the office, knock on the door, and wait for the managers to respond. Then they would conscientiously try to help him.

These two styles represent two different philosophies of sponsorship, and it is difficult to say whether one is better than the other. The crucial question is which style is the more comfortable for sponsor and resident. Individual preferences vary. Some residents don't want the manager to become actively involved in their lives; others like him to assume a larger role in their everyday living. The depressed suicidal patient who goes into a residence with the boardinghouse-style philosophy may not always announce the fact that he has an immediate, pressing problem. If the policy is to wait for the resident to show up at a time of crisis, the wait may be too long.

The resident may be approached effectively by talking with him while the sponsor works or by inviting him to work alongside the sponsor. Some of Kent's most rewarding contacts with staff took place as they watered the lawn together or as he helped to refill a Coke machine. First comes contact, a personal human contact, and then may come a personal contract. This contract centers on the resident's promise to tell the staff before he does anything harmful to himself. A verbal contract is especially valuable when a resident is depressed or suicidal. It marks a mutual willingness to be open about suicide and the establishment of mutual trust. There need be no worry about putting the idea of suicide into a patient's mind; if the patient is suicidal, the idea is already there. Talking about suicide with the resident and getting it "out on the table" (just like bringing racial differences to the surface) is good policy.

Giving Information

Part of the art of being a sponsor or manager is to offer information and to repeat it often enough so that it is remembered. In some places roommates as well as sponsors were careful to make sure that Kent knew the address of the residence or that he had in writing on his person at all times the name of the facility, the address, the phone number, and the manager's name. One sponsor came to Kent's room and said, "There's a guy who may pace at night but don't let it upset you. He paces every night." She was warning him and thus helping him to recognize and accept conditions as they were and to make reasonable plans in his world.

Depression

For a depressed person, keeping up the depression takes a bit of work. A number of factors make it difficult or easy for a person to stay depressed. In the first place, most depressions do not consist of a single continuous "low." Everyone, even a severely depressed person, has mood cycles. One day he may feel slightly better than he did the day before. He wakes up that morning feeling somewhat more active; he wants to get out and socialize. When a depressed person feels even this incremental desire for activity, there should be opportunities waiting for him: stairs to climb, phones to answer, wastebaskets to empty, people to talk to, and work and play to engage his attention. If the opportunities are available, he may take advantage of them. Merely sitting for a day, doing absolutely nothing, brings profound changes to body and mind. Kent found himself becoming gloomy and constipated, his mind becoming dull and his body lazy. Without oppressive pushing, the more a depressed person can be encouraged to move about and to act constructively and purposefully, the less chance he has of sliding deeper into depression.

Besides the mood cycles, Kent felt cycles of (1) being smothered by people whom he wished would get off his back and (2) being abandoned by them. In one situation a sponsor invited him to church and then repeated the invitation later, but when Sunday came the project had apparently been forgotten or abandoned. Another sponsor promised to bring him a television set on Monday, but when Monday came, no TV set appeared. Kent was able to tell himself that he didn't care, that perhaps they didn't feel he was ready, that the time was not exactly right, or that they had forgotten. Whatever the reason, he felt abandoned. The sponsor needs acute sensitivity to pick up these moods. But most important is the sponsor's need to be honest in his relationships with residents. Depressed people (like many other mentally disturbed people) are quick to sense artificiality.

When a resident feels "down," the tendency is to tell him to feel better, perhaps to try to joke or kid him out of his mood. A truly depressed person is often prompted by such an approach to withdraw further, feeling that he is not understood. His response, in turn, may arouse frustration or anger in those who are trying to help him. An alternative approach is to accept the reality that everybody has a right to feel bad. A man's depression should be respected and honored, just as his joy is respected and honored. It often helps simply to sit quietly with him, letting him know that his feelings are being shared. An offer of companionship, an invitation to accompany the sponsor on his work rounds or in play activity, when appropriate, can be meaningful to the depressed person. The objective is to involve him in activities with other people to the degree that he can accept.

The principle that one should not directly oppose an opponent's strength holds sway in judo and karate. It is better to move with the force, deflecting it slightly. If one avoids fighting against another person's depression, if one even shares it and uses it to build closeness and trust that will help in guiding the person out of his despair, then the force of the depression is working for, not against, the helper. The principle is the same as in the martial arts.

Weekends are very different from weekdays in aftercare residences. They are usually even more boring. Kent was placed in two of the facilities on a Friday afternoon and then had almost nothing to do until Monday morning. Facilities with an inactive weekend program might better admit people only on Mondays and Tuesdays, when they can be plunged immediately into the activity program.

Finally, it should be remembered that depressive persons are self-centered, even selfish. As they start to feel better, some have such strong needs for a sense of self-worth that they seek confirmation by asking the helper to give them his most precious possession. If he agrees, his act means to them that they are worth even more than the thing he relinquishes. The most valuable possession varies: it may be time, or privacy, or a special television show, or a family relationship. Whatever it is, the depressed person seems able to sense it, as a starving man unfailingly detects the smell of food in the air. That precious item, however, should not be given to the depressed person. Instead, he should be offered information and unlimited evidence of concern. The information should tell him how he can gain people's respect through work and decent behavior. The concern should be in terms of interest and a sincere desire to help. The depressed person wants self-respect, self-confidence, a self that is worth keeping alive. The most important lesson for him to learn is that he has to earn something that he really wants.

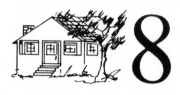# 8 GENERAL RECOMMENDATIONS

What suggestions can be made to improve life for both residents and staff in aftercare facilities? These facilities may be an important stepping-stone in the mental hospital patient's progress back to the community. Therefore his experience in the facility is often a primary determinant of the future course of his life. Kent's and Summers's experiences have given us an intensive awareness of the influences, both gross and subtle, to which the resident is exposed and thus make it possible for us to offer suggestions and recommendations for improvement of the facilities and enhancement of their ability to smooth the transition from patient to community member.

Graded Facilities

First, we suggest that aftercare facilities be grouped or graded according to orientation and program. Some patients want a permanent home; others want sheltered protection for the moment until they are ready to move out on their own; still others need training for independent living. The different categories require different programs, and it is absurd to expect facilities to mount expensive training programs that will meet the needs of only one of these categories. Yet it is callous to provide no training for those who are motivated to live independently.

One solution might be to have specialized facilities. Residents could then move from one facility to another in an effort to realize the goal of independence. Residences that cater to settled, permanent guests could provide appropriate activities and enjoy a steady income. Those that help the resident toward self-sufficiency could charge more for the extra training facilities and for providing training cooperatives in the community. Furthermore, the latter type of establishment could receive some sort of bonus for each graduating resident who successfully "makes it" in the community for a specified period of time. Thus the programs in all facilities would not be weighted toward keeping a passive, long-term clientele.

Discharge Patterns

Patients who leave hospitals and aftercare facilities move from "success" (i.e., discharge) to the bottom rung of a new social ladder. It is at this critical juncture, when a depressed person is trying to establish a new identity in the community and when he most needs social support, that he is left completely on his own. We believe experiments should be undertaken to explore the possibility of discharging patients and residents in pairs or larger groups, instead of one by one. They would then have available a mutual social support system as they encounter the stresses of adjusting to the community.

An additional impetus for success on the outside might be a kind of "graduating" ceremony, a farewell party or the like, at the time of discharge from the residence. When Kent left the residences in which he had been placed he felt a sense of anticlimax; people seemed not to care, and perhaps did not even know, that he was about to leave. A ward or residence celebration would send the departing member off with the warm good wishes and positive expectations of his peers. A parting gift of donated money might reinforce movement toward independence and, however small, would be a welcome practical adjunct at a time it is most likely to be needed.

We should not discount the fact that for many people the sheltered life in a hospital or an aftercare facility may be strongly preferred to an isolated existence in a faceless society. Freedom may be gladly given up in exchange for protection and absence of responsibility. And it is not only the patient who feels this way. The community life of a hospital ward or in a board-and-care home offers to some staff members variety, purpose, and a deep level of human contact rarely available elsewhere in our society. It is the kind of environment that draws and holds them, even for patently difficult and low-paying jobs.

It may be unreasonable to expect people to want to leave a

home, a job, friends, a daily routine, a leisurely noncompetitive life style, and a familiar community in order to divide his time between a boring job and a lonely apartment. Keep in mind that residents left in a home are likely to lose touch immediately with those who make a go of it in the wider community, but that they hear over and over again the sad tales of those who were unsuccessful on the outside and had to return. Most residents are offered no help in setting themselves up on the outside or in developing skills and habits that will sustain independent living. Actually, they are "punished" for leaving the hospital or aftercare facility by a cutback in welfare benefits at precisely the time when their need of resources is the most compelling.

The ultimate solution to the problem of pulling people out of institutions and enabling them to establish themselves successfully is the difficult, long-term process of making the society into which they emerge a more attractive and meaningful one.

Staff and Resident Organization

Staff members in aftercare facilities usually find their roles defined by tasks. Cooking, managing, handling finances, providing recreation, maintaining good living conditions, and the like are the necessary dimensions of staff roles. We would like to see each staff member assigned to a small group of residents. Whatever his task-defined role, he would meet with his particular group of residents once or twice a week, and he would be responsible for talking briefly with each of them on an individual basis each day. In turn, the residents would be organized into pairs or trios with the assignment of meeting briefly with their partners each day. The exchange could be facilitated by encouraging assigned partners to sit together at meals. Newcomers could be introduced into the system immediately upon entry, providing a reciprocal information source and a chance to be helpful.

Psychological Inoculation

It is important to be aware of a resident's career, from newcomer to interim status, to full membership in the aftercare community, and finally to termination. It may be possible to practice a kind of psychological "inoculation" into and through the various stages. In part, the impact of the loss of newcomer status, or the fear of leaving, lies in the unexpectedness and the lack of understanding of what is being experienced. If we can forewarn ex-patients of the experiences they are likely to have, and give them a conceptual framework for handling them (these are natural steps in the orderly, progressive return to community life), we can reduce the probability of their encountering setbacks. What is expected and natural becomes more controllable and less traumatic. Indeed, the fact that we can foresee what the resident is likely to experience makes our other predictions and suggestions more weighty. Many patients and ex-patients feel strongly that professionals have no real sense of what they go through. The suggested approach would signify that we have listened to a resident's accounts of his experience and have used the knowledge to build our understanding of and our credibility with him.

We also advocate a modified educator-consultant role for after-care managers, and for mental health professionals in general, because such a role would permit the client to share in controlling the interaction. Moreover, it would emphasize the importance of timing the interaction to meet the felt needs of the client. We believe, however, that the consultant must actively seek to establish an initial relationship of trust and mutual confidence so that the client feels free to seek the consultant out and to respond honestly in his interactions with the consultant. A consultant can be used effectively (or used at all) only if the client perceives him to be trustworthy and helpful.

The initial cementing of an interpersonal tie is particularly important for a suicidal client. The suicidal person needs to know that at least one knowledgeable, sympathetic person stands ready to cooperate in his efforts to achieve a worthwhile life.

Courtesy and Respect

Research experience in mental disorders in several cultures and subcultures has impressed us less by the differences among humans than by their similarities. The category really makes no difference, whether Japanese, black, Jew, mentally disturbed, suicidal, healthy, patient, staff member, or aftercare resident. Each must be understood in relation to his setting. Often what appears at first to be strange, or "crazy," behavior begins to make sense when we come to understand the situation context in which the behavior occurs.

Too often we slip into the misconception that a helping relationship is confined to the hours of formal therapy in an office. The greeting a staff member offers a resident in the hall on the way to his office may make the resident's day or undermine it. A resident may see the aftercare management as his sole channel for bringing about a major change in his medication or residence or economic situation. It is an awesome responsibility that our psychiatric system and the residents themselves place on residential aftercare sponsors.

Listening to the resident and taking him seriously is therapeutic in itself. Finding out what life is like in his immediate situation is at least as important as learning about his early childhood and his current adult personality configuration. Furthermore, when we ask the right questions and he finds we are genuinely interested in what is going on in his living facility, the resident is much more likely to give us coherent information than he does when we probe his psyche for depth material. The patient himself is the expert on the setting in which he lives. Situational variables are not superficial elements; instead, they are of vast importance in determining how we behave, regardless of background or diagnosis or personality pattern.

Acts of courtesy and respect convey a message of worth which is meaningful and necessary to all of us. We constantly monitor and evaluate such messages from others, whether or not we are aware of the process. For the depressed, suicidal person, for the institutionalized, stigmatized person, these communications are vitally important. In the preceding pages we have documented some of the behavioral language in which these messages are couched.

We must not let our formal training and professionalism set us apart from and "above" our clients, residents, and patients; we cannot afford to forget the simple lesson of the value of common humanness. Lives depend on it and are saved by it.

APPENDIX

SOCIAL SERVICES

REPORTS AND
SUMMARIES

Plan for community living

I. Identifying data: Non-service connected. Birth date   9-28-40
    Next of kin/guardian ____Sharon Kent (wife)_____
    Address ___2228 9th St. North, St. Petersburg, Fla.__ Phone _____
    Notified of plan and placement? _Yes_____
    Wife's maiden name _Sharon Kay_____

II. Disposition:Discharge____OPT-SC ___ OPT-NSC _X_ NBC ___
    Home _____ CNH _____N.H. _____B&C _X__Other _____

III. Finances: Sources and amounts
    VA compensation ___VA pension ___Retirement ___A&A __
    Social security_____ATD _____ Other _Savings___
    Mailed where?_____
    Patient's funds? ___$420_____
    Cost of care _$198_ Personal allowance _____ Paid by _____
    Competent for VA?_Yes_____ Legal status? _____

IV. Patient:

    1. Reason for placement

        Hospitalization no longer indicated. Pt. planning on going to
        school and/or finding work. Considering going to Woodbury
        College in Los Angeles.

    2. Description of patient (behavior, appearance, personality
        moods)

        Small, meek, slumped-over young man. Sometimes tearful
        and uncommunicative but appears fairly alert. Keeps to
        himself. Occasionally depressed and preoccupied.

3. Psychiatric problems (kind of supervision needed)

Depressed, passive, one suicidal attempt. Needs firm encouragement to socialize and participate in activities.

4. Physical disabilities, problems (need glasses, dentures, hearing aid, etc.)

Wears glasses, takes care of himself fairly well.

5. What medication is prescribed and how is it to be handled?
Physician: <u>   Crockett   </u>

Elavil 25 mg. bid.

6. Medical clearance (result and date of tests)

7. Special dietary problems, needs

V. <u>Plans</u>:

1. Attitudes of patient and family

Married sister has little contact with patient. Wife is seeking divorce which precipitated suicide attempt. Patient apathetic.

2. Work potential

He should be able to go to work. Wants to be a writer. Is seriously considering going to college.

3. Hobbies, church, social activities

4. Name and address of friends willing to help patient

Larry Evans (friend), address unknown.

5. Type of sponsor and supervision needed

Encouragement, support, to get out and socialize, to find work or get schooling in which he can get personal satisfaction.

IV. Additional recommendations: Who will do the follow-up?

Keith Froehlich

BIBLIOGRAPHY

Alkire, A. A., Pearman, H. E., and McCarthy, C. D. Pairing of patient-sponsor to reduce conflict costs in home care of patients diagnosed as schizophrenic. *Journal of Clinical Psychology, 22* (Oct.), 472-476, 1966.

Braginsky, Benjamin M., et al. *Methods of Madness.* New York: Holt, Rinehart and Winston, 1969.

Carhill, K. G. A community placement program for state hospital patients. *Mental Hygiene, 51*(2), 261-265, 1967.

Chase, C., Gross, S., Hanna, B., Israel, L., and Woods, E. Board and care — structure, sponsor and orientation: a descriptive study of large board and care homes used by Brentwood Hospital. Master of Social Welfare thesis, *University of California,* Los Angeles, 1970.

Cunningham, M. K., Botwinik, W., Dolson, J., and Weickert, A. A. Community placement of released mental patients: a five-year study. *Social Work, 14*(1), 54-61, 1969.

David, J. E. Family care of the mentally ill in Norway. *American Journal of Psychiatry, 119* (Aug.), 154-158, 1962.

Dumont, M. P., and Aldrich, C. K. Family care after a thousand years: a crisis in the tradition of St. Dymphna. *American Journal of Psychiatry, 119* (Aug.), 116-121, 1962.

Farberow, Normal L., et al. An eight-year survey of hospital suicides. *Life-Threatening Behavior, 1,* 184-202, 1971.

Friedman, I., von Mering, O., and Hinko, E. N. Intermittent patienthood. *Archives of General Psychiatry, 14* (April), 386-392, 1966.

Goffman, E. *Asylums.* New York: Doubleday, 1961.

Gurel, L., and Lorei, T. Hospital and community ratings of psychopathology as predictors of employment and readmission. *Journal of Consulting and Clinical Psychology, 39*(2), 286-291, 1972.

Kemp, Joan. Social characteristics of chronic mental patients. Unpublished MS. UCLA School of Social Work, Brentwood VA Hospital, December, 1972.

Laing, R. D. *Sanity, Madness and the Family.* London: Tavistock, 1961.

Lamb, H. R., and Goertzel, V. Discharged mental patients: are they really in the community? *Archives of General Psychiatry, 24* (Jan.), 29-34, 1971.

_____. The demise of the state hospital: a premature obituary? *Archives of General Psychiatry, 26* (June), 489-495, 1972.

Lamb, H. Richard, and associates. *Community Survival for Long-Term Patients.* San Francisco: Jossey-Bass, 1967.

Lee, D. T. Family care: selection and prediction. *American Journal of Psychiatry, 120* (Dec.), 561-566, 1963.

Linn, M. W., Brown, C. W., Miller, N. D., Thompson, R. G., and Wathan, R. L. Family care: a therapeutic tool for the chronic mental patient. *Archives of General Psychiatry, 15* (Sept.), 276-278, 1966.

Linn, M. W., Caffey, E. M., Klett, C. James, and Hogarty, G. Hospital versus community (foster) care for psychiatric patients. Unpublished MS. Veterans Administration Cooperative Study, Washington, D.C., 1975.

Lorei, T., and Gurel, L. Use of a biographical inventory to predict schizophrenics' posthospital employment and readmission. *Journal of Consulting and Clinical Psychology, 38*(2), 238-243, 1972.

Lyle, C. M. and Trail, O. A study of psychiatric patients in foster homes. *Social Work, 6*(1), 82-88, 1961.

McCarthy, C. D., Alkire, A. A., and Pearman, H. E. Factor analysis of conflict areas occurring in home placement of patients diagnosed as schizophrenic. *Journal of Clinical Psychology, 21*(1), 85-89, 1965.

Morrissey, J. R. Family care for the mentally ill: a neglected therapeutic resource. *Social Service Review, 39*(1), 63-71, 1965.

Reynolds, David K. The board-and-care home: a resident's view. Paper presented at the Symposium on Community Mental Health, Los Angeles, California, 1975.

_____. *Morita Psychotherapy.* Berkeley, Los Angeles, and London: University of California Press, 1976.

Reynolds, David K., and Farberow, Norman L. *Suicide: Inside and Out.* Berkeley, Los Angeles, and London: University of California Press, 1976.

Ullmann, L. P., and Berkman, V. C. Efficacy of placement of neuropsychiatric patients in family care. *Archives of General Psychiatry, 1* (Sept.), 273-274, 1959a.

_____. Judgments of outcome of home-care placement from psychological material. *Journal of Clinical Psychology, 51*(1), 1959b.

Ullmann, L. P., Berkman, V. C. and Hamister, R. C. Psychological reports related to behavior and benefit of placement in home care. *Journal of Clinical Psychology, 14*(3), 254-259, 1958.

INDEX